The Body Knows... How to Stay Young

For Audrey!
Stay young!
Caroline ♡

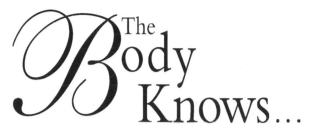

The Body Knows...

How to Stay Young

HEALTHY-AGING SECRETS
FROM A MEDICAL INTUITIVE

CAROLINE SUTHERLAND

HAY HOUSE, INC.
Carlsbad, California • New York City
London • Sydney • Johannesburg
Vancouver • Hong Kong • New Delhi

Published and distributed in the United States by: Hay House, Inc.:
www.hayhouse.com • *Published and distributed in Australia by:* Hay
House Australia Pty. Ltd.: www.hayhouse.com.au • *Published and
distributed in the United Kingdom by:* Hay House UK, Ltd.: www.
hayhouse.co.uk • *Published and distributed in the Republic of South
Africa by:* Hay House SA (Pty), Ltd.: www.hayhouse.co.za • *Distributed
in Canada by:* Raincoast: www.raincoast.com • *Published in India by:*
Hay House Publishers India: www.hayhouse.co.in

Editorial supervision: Jill Kramer • *Design:* Tricia Breidenthal

Library of Congress Cataloging-in-Publication Data

Sutherland, Caroline M.
   The body knows-- how to stay young : healthy-aging secrets from a
medical intuitive / Caroline Sutherland.
     p. cm.
   ISBN-13: 978-1-4019-2024-1 (tradepaper) 1. Aging--Prevention--
Popular works. 2. Longevity--Popular works. I. Title.
   RA776.75.S89 2008
   613.2--dc22   2008003825

ISBN: 978-1-4019-2024-1

11 10 09 08   4 3 2 1
1st edition, July 2008

Printed in the United States of America

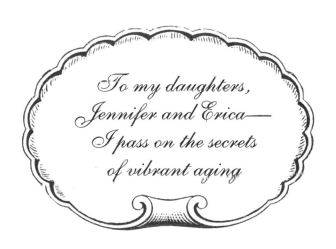

To my daughters,
Jennifer and Erica—
I pass on the secrets
of vibrant aging

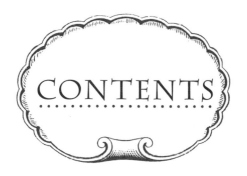

CONTENTS

PART IV: Ignite Your Passion

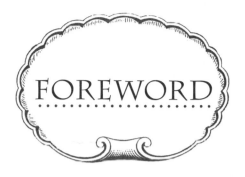

FOREWORD

You, dear reader, have no idea how blessed you are to have this book in your hands. I longed for something just like it when I entered menopause 30 years ago—a guide that would give me precise details on how to maintain my health and have vibrant energy as I grew older, as well as giving me options so that I could help create my own optimal program.

I've been a Caroline Sutherland fan ever since the first moment I met her in the 1990s. In fact, she fulfilled a dream of mine. At our first meeting, Caroline looked at me, clearly saw my deficiencies and nutritional needs, and on the spot designed a special food plan for my particular body. I called it the "You Diet" as opposed to the "Cookie-Cutter Diet," or one size for everyone. I felt understood for the first time.

Like many people, over the years I tried all the systems: raw food, macrobiotic, vegetarian, fruitarian, deny yourself this, deny yourself that, only eat this one item. I followed each one for a period of time and never felt my best. I certainly did not fit in to those "one size fits all" regimens.

I had long been aware that most diet or nutrition books were written by people who had physical problems and discovered a way to heal their own bodies. They then wrote volumes that said, in effect, "Everyone has to follow these rules in order to get well or thin." Well, every body is not the same as every other body on the planet. We are all individuals, so one food plan cannot work for every person.

Caroline Sutherland's first book, *The Body "Knows": How to Tune In to Your Body and Improve Your Health,* has been invaluable to thousands of men and women, including myself. However, as we age, we have special requirements for keeping ourselves in tip-top shape. Society as a whole has never before had such a large aging population, nor have we been confronted with the enormous amounts of junk and processed foods available to us.

Wheat, dairy, and sugar—especially high-fructose corn syrup—seem to be everywhere and in everything we consume. We're now in the middle of a national experiment in mainlining glucose. Our bodies aren't meant to handle this onslaught and are breaking down at such a rapid rate that medicine has had to learn how to keep alive those whom the Western diet has made so sick.

Our reliance on chemicals, both in foods and in medicine, is destroying our health. We must turn away from them if we are to regain and maintain our health, yet doing so requires special knowledge and information.

That's where Caroline Sutherland comes in. *The Body Knows . . . How to Stay Young: Healthy-Aging Secrets from a Medical Intuitive* takes us to the next step. I read this book in one sitting, enthralled to find such a storehouse of information, filled with everything I was looking for and so much more.

I'm now in my 80s. I am very healthy and have lots of good energy, and I want to keep it that way until the day I leave the planet. I don't believe that we have to become ill in order to die. Rather, I believe it is our birthright to enjoy vibrant health as long as we're alive. Caroline shows us how to arrest the body's breakdown process and then move into the repair and regeneration mode.

All you have to do is meet Caroline in person and you'll be amazed by how incredibly healthy she is. This is exactly the type of person whose advice I want to follow for nutritional guidance. I feel honored to have her as my guide and mentor in this exciting journey. I'm so excited that you have this opportunity, too. When you follow the suggestions in this book, you'll be well on *your* way to perfect aging and vibrant wellness.

Here's to great health for you and me into our 100s. We can do it!

— **Louise L. Hay**
San Diego, California

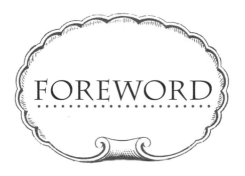

FOREWORD

I think we all start out in life "intuitively" a little skeptical of "intuition"—and for no particular reason other than the fact that we really don't understand how it works. For me it was a gender issue: From day one, I was told that it was only women who had intuition. They were actually born with it! It was in their genes! It was always referred to as "a woman's intuition" or sometimes as "a mother's intuition" but never, ever "a man's intuition." It just wasn't kosher for a man to be intuitive, at least not in Kansas City, Missouri, in the '40s and '50s. Hard facts, mathematics, physics, chemistry, and nuts and bolts were our male heritage, and they didn't come easy. But I can tell you that when hard facts were pitted against a woman's intuition in those days (or perhaps these days as well), there was no contest—women's intuition won, hands down.

During my adolescent years of intellectual rebellion, I decided to get to the bottom of this gender discrimination. I went straight to Merriam-Webster's dictionary, which defined *intuition* as "the power or faculty of gaining direct knowledge or cognition without evident rational thought and inference." Now I was fascinated. Did women somehow have a hotline to direct knowledge and/or cognition, without rational thought or inference, while men were forever cursed with the labor of logic and reason to make sense out of our universe? I was now greedily beginning to experience "intuition envy."

Medical school did little to resolve my conflict. Rational differential diagnoses, systematic treatment protocols, precise medical calibrations, and rigorously defined outcome statistics were the order of the day. "Institution" had been substituted for "intuition." The subject of intuition was nowhere to be found in the curriculum—even though there were three women in my class who, by virtue of their gifted gender intuitiveness, could no doubt have elaborated on the innate sensitivity of human beings to diagnose themselves without benefit of stethoscope or tongue blades! Of course this was way back in 1971, when dinosaurs still walked the streets of Little Rock, Arkansas, and the age of intuitive enlightenment had yet to dawn over the entrenched medical mainstays of diagnosing and prescribing scientifically by the numbers.

In a real-world private practice of medicine, however, everything changes. You do everything you can by the book, and then one day you realize that "evident rational thought and inference" don't always win the day. Sometimes your intuition (or your patient's) emerges as the more appropriate answer and seems much more effective than evidence-based research. This can be especially true when the numbers on the laboratory analysis of a blood test simply do not match the patient who sits in front of you. So somehow you wake up one morning realizing that much of what you do is intuitive . . . and it works!

One of my favorite celebrity doctors, Andrew Weil, M.D., contends that the body can heal itself given the opportunity to do so. The real impact of medicine, he reasons, is not to cure, but to reduce the pathological agent of destruction to a low enough level for the body's natural defenses to take over the job of healing. As one of my patients pointed out, "No one ever died of a blood-serum antibiotic deficiency."

If the body can heal itself from disease under the right conditions, can it also intuitively know how to stay young? There's no question in my mind that the body knows to respond to the opportunity to maintain its youth. I know that because it is this exact intuitive sense of aging that has driven thousands of patients to my office over the last 14 years—not pain, not cancer, not a fractured hip, but the undeniable sense that things aren't what they used to be and "I want my life back."

Ironically, many of these patients admit to me that they know intuitively what they should or shouldn't be doing to stay young, but they *simply don't trust their own intuition.* Why? Well, in part because medical science has conditioned us to accept the ravages of aging as the natural sequence of events and indoctrinated us to believe that whatever goes wrong can be "fixed" with a pill or a shot or a scalpel.

The other part of the equation is our own stubborn reluctance to give up even a single minute of our valuable time that could be used for garnering money, power, and prestige to listen to our body's plea for help. And finally, there are those who reach a certain stage in life and, for lack of a better phrase, "just plain give up." They feel it's too late, they're too old, and there are no answers left for them—or, worse yet, it just isn't worth the trouble for them to take charge of their health.

Please put all these negative excuses out of your mind and listen to your body. There is an incredible future ahead of you, no matter what age or stage in life you find yourself. If you're thinking, *That's easy for you to say, doctor,* you're absolutely right! I have seen, felt, heard, and read the responses to these principles of rejuvenation as outlined here by Caroline Sutherland, day after day, patient after patient, for the last 14 years. These "Healthy-Aging Secrets from a Medical Intuitive," which are so wonderfully illustrated with life stories of amazing restoration, are inspirational guidelines that have universal application.

Caroline's writing is warm, personal, and compassionate, just like Caroline is in person. You'll find a resonance in her research that will resurrect and liberate your body's struggle to find youthful expression. Today, this minute, the options are here on these pages, in black and white. It's no longer conjecture—the science is real, the research is convincing and validating, and the results are astounding. My prescription for you is Caroline's well-written invitation to optimize your health. I know that as you read and discover her enlightening and empowering insights into an intuitively guided rejuvenation, you'll savor the incredible gift of intuition, just as I have.

— **Joe Filbeck, M.D.**
San Diego, California

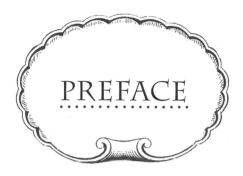

PREFACE

Thanks to my experience as a medical intuitive, and from the thousands of readings I've done over the years, I believe that the body has the capacity to repair at any age. It doesn't matter if we're in our 60s, 70s, or 80s, our bodies "know" what to do.

The body is like a great house with lots of possibilities. Since it's tough and has a firm foundation, all it needs is a fresh coat of paint, a little tinkering here and there, and to have the furniture rearranged—and voilà! It will be as good as new.

In *The Body Knows . . . How to Stay Young*, I'll illustrate how we can all slow down the aging process to the point that we move into repair and regeneration mode. Then as we progress in years, we can live actively; attractively; healthfully; vibrantly; and, above all, passionately.

My motivation in writing this book is to make it personal and human. This isn't some dry tome, but rather a resource that everyone can use and relate to. In it, I share stories about the people I meet each day and how they're coping with their health and aging challenges. I offer insights into my own healing journey as well, including the steps I've personally taken to slow down the biological passage of time.

I don't pay much attention to folks who say that aging is a wonderful process to be revered. After all, they say, wine improves with age, and moldy old cheese is such a delicacy. Bah, humbug! Sure, there are some great benefits that come with growing older, such as the joy of being a grandparent, reduced rates at movies, and free rides on public transport, but I'm not about to compare my life with a lump of Limburger . . . no thanks. I'm more interested in enhancing the possibilities.

Who wants to be in a nursing home or spend their days being pushed around in a wheelchair? Not me. When it comes to aging, I'll vote for good vision, strong bones, sharp memory, vitality, sparkle, freedom from pain, and wisdom to boot! Unfortunately, in my work as a medical intuitive, I see so many people who are way out of balance and aging fast—they turn old before their time.

Just the other day I met a woman who's the same age as I am, but she looked ten years older. She was overweight, lacking energy, obviously in pain, and surrounded by a lot of sadness. I'm very concerned for people like this, which is why I teach others how to slow down the aging process and capitalize on the years they have yet to live to make them their best.

After 25 years of working intuitively with thousands of people, I believe that there are four secrets of vibrant aging, and I'm so excited to share them with you in these pages:

1. Stop the body breakdown.
2. Regenerate and repair the body.
3. Balance hormones.
4. Ignite your passion.

Thus, that's how I've divided this book. Working with these four principles increases the body's capacity for maintenance and repair—*not* reproduction and cell division, which increase the risk of cancer and other age-related degenerative diseases. In each chapter, I discuss important ways to alter the pace of the aging process. Please note that some chapters are longer than others, but that doesn't mean that any one concept is more important than another. It's all part of one big healthy-aging concert, in which each instrument plays in harmony with the others.

This book is designed to help you become all that you were intended to be. Your purpose is to reach your full potential and to fulfill your destiny before you die.

So with that goal in mind, let's take the journey into new territory: the terrain of vibrant aging. Grab your map and your compass, and we'll reach that destination together.

PART I
· · · · · · · · · · · ·

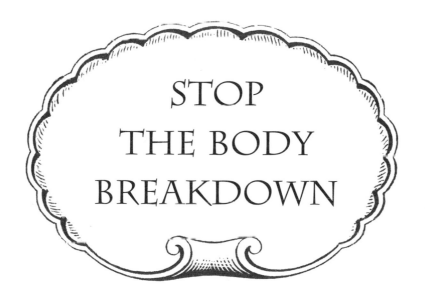

STOP
THE BODY
BREAKDOWN

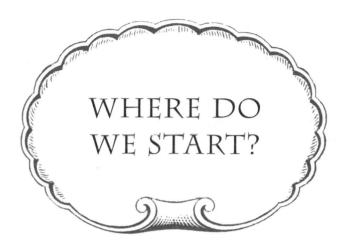

CHAPTER 1

WHERE DO
WE START?

· ·

This year I turned 64. Where did the time go? I have lived, loved, and watched my children grow up; and now here I am, a grandmother, and aging with a capital "A."

I remember sitting in the backseat of the family Plymouth not that long ago as my mother drove my sister, my brother, and me to our swimming lessons in a neighboring town. The year was 1954, and I was ten years old.

The car windows were open, so I could smell the summer air blowing over our three fresh, tanned, and freckled faces. I looked over at my mother as she steered us along on the bumpy road, and I noticed that her upper arms began to jiggle. *What's that?* I wondered. *My arms don't jiggle. I'll never let my arms jiggle!* Well, guess what? Aging is inevitable, bringing with it jiggly arms, mottled hands, and sagging and sinking this and that. But do we have to die of old age and chronic disease? No, I don't believe we do.

I'm a medical intuitive, which means that I have the ability to "see" beyond the normal levels of perception into subtle levels below. I got my start as an allergy-testing technician in the early 1980s, working for medical doctors and naturopathic physicians, but I didn't come to this work a healthy woman. In fact, I had the early warning signs of multiple sclerosis in 1983—including numbness and tingling in the arms and hands, memory loss, balance problems, bumping into tables and doorways, depression, and other seemingly unrelated symptoms. Then, by a stroke of good fortune, my own family physician referred me to a doctor who specialized in environmental medicine. It was discovered that all my symptoms were related to environmental factors such as food intolerance, airborne allergies, chemical sensitivities, yeast-related issues, and hormone imbalances.

Within a month of dietary modifications and specific treatment, I was symptom free . . . and I've remained so ever since. Now, 25 years later, I believe that the lifestyle changes I made and the regimen I've been following have set me on a course to age in a healthy manner. And it's time to pass on this information to you.

In a clinical setting, I was involved in the assessment and treatment of more than 55,000 individuals, thus honing the gift of medical intuition. I could actually see things in the patients and sense their bodies' breakdown. For more than two decades, I've had the privilege of working with many thousands of people, and I'm very passionate about what I do. Helping men and women become healthy is my purpose and my destiny, which I clearly learned as I almost died. . . .

In 1995, I was making a left turn on a busy country road. As I waited for oncoming traffic to pass, I looked in my rearview mirror and saw a blue pickup truck approaching very quickly. I was hit with a "smack" from behind, and all I could feel was that I wasn't "done"—I was about to die, but I hadn't completed my purpose on Earth. I had never experienced such a deep feeling of sadness. But there was no time to reflect on that, as I was immediately taken to a plane of existence that I'd call "infinity." This was a place without boundaries or horizons, just brilliant light. It felt like the beat or pulse of all existence, or an infinite heartbeat, and there appeared to be a rhythm or order to all of life. I was shown that life was short and very precious, that our time was to be spent caring for other people and the planet, waking up, and becoming conscious: fulfilling our unique destiny before it was too late.

At that level I was even able to communicate with souls who had obviously been born and then died, and who appeared to be waiting to reenter the physical. I had the unique opportunity of communicating with these souls, who told me telepathically that they "would give anything to be in a physical body." According to them, I was to feel fortunate to have a body and be of service; these were great privileges that should be treated with the highest reverence.

There was no time to pursue the conversation further, because all of a sudden I was back in my car. I was gripping the steering wheel and powering through a grassy ditch, only to come to a full stop just inches away from a road sign. What a miracle.

That very-near-death experience was a wake-up call and a pivotal moment for me. Since that day, I've become a teacher (a zealot, really) encouraging others to get on board, get healthy, and get their individual jobs done before their time to leave the planet arrives.

I guarantee that none of us wants to have a life review and see that our time has been wasted. So in order to have the vitality to complete our purpose, we must turn back the aging clock and restore health and vitality to our bodies.

Inner Direction on Aging Vibrantly

When you look around at folks who are over the age of 70, I'll bet you notice that they don't look very good. If you have elderly parents, your daily thought may even be, *Dear God, just don't let me end up like this.*

I'm with you. I'm very interested to see people in their 70s, 80s, and 90s who are vivacious, energetic, and fully engaged in life . . . sadly, they're few and far between. Yet with almost $50 billion spent annually on supplements and alternative treatments, people are finally waking up to the fact that good health is priceless.

My path in catching the wellness wave was shown to me spiritually when I took a trip to England in 1986. At that time, I'd been working in environmental medicine for almost three years and was ready to take some advanced courses.

It was Easter week when I arrived, and I had the chance to attend some of the services at Salisbury Cathedral near Southampton. I walked in, sat down, and perused the church bulletin. There I spotted the well-known story of Noah and the ark, and when I got to the end of it, a still, small voice inside my head said: *Read it again.*

I looked at the story: ". . . and God said to Noah . . . the people laughed at Noah . . . the animals two by two . . . and the floods came . . . ," and so on. When I finished, my inner voice gently told me to read it yet again. So I did, this time taking careful note of each of the elements. I especially focused on the part about people questioning Noah about his idea of building an ark in the middle of the desert with no body of water in sight.

When I was done, I stayed quiet, listening for the next piece of guidance to come. *You, too, will be building an ark,* my inner voice told me. *People will question you, even judge or mock you, but you must keep your focus. One day your ark will float, and many people will want to come aboard. Do not give up. Show the way to others about the importance of becoming healthy. Stay steadfast and strong.*

Just like me, you're also building an ark—that of your own life and spiritual purpose. So stay focused, listen to your inner guidance, and come aboard with your health goals.

Personally, at 50 I didn't see any real signs of aging— I even wore a backless dress for my 50th birthday party. There was nary a wrinkle or a line to be seen upon me, and life was grand. Then, two years later, my daughter and I went to the south of France to visit my brother, who was there with his family on sabbatical from his university job. It was a marvelous experience, and the food was marvelous, too!

I returned several pounds heavier, with a little dimpled pouchy stomach that I didn't have before. And almost overnight, my skin wasn't as tight and elastic as it used to be. These were the first signs that I was aging.

I purchased some new skin cream from my aesthetician, was able to lose the weight I'd gained, and life went on. The next development came several years later when my waistline began to expand, with no apparent letup in sight. This time I couldn't seem to whittle it down, no matter how little I ate or how much I exercised. That's when the universe brought me my next step: I discovered a low-carbohydrate diet and retrieved my waistline. Saved again!

Then, seemingly out of nowhere, the next little fun wrinkle (no pun intended) to appear came in the form of hot flashes, night sweats, anxiety, and overreacting meltdowns that had me concerned. Enter a wonderful holistic medical doctor in Arizona who prepared individually tailored homeopathic hormone drops that nipped all of those symptoms in the bud for a number of years. Yet the portcullis came down once more.

What now? Just as I've always believed it would, the universe delivered again. When I happened to see a TV program about natural hormone balancing, I knew it was the next step. As I'd just turned 60, my medical doctor had been encouraging me to try natural or bioidentical hormone balancing for my menopausal issues, and this show seemed to be a sign from the universe to proceed. I was ready to get on board, and I'm so glad I did. Four years later, I feel as if the hands of time are moving much more slowly.

Vi and Dorothy

I spend several months each year in a beautiful condo complex right on the ocean. There are many elderly people who live here; in fact, the place is something of a retirement home. But imagine going to sleep at night with the sound of the sea at your feet, and the seagulls calling out to you in the morning. It's heaven! No wonder people want to live here until the ambulance comes (which it does quite often) to carry them off to the morgue or the hospital.

I figured that this neighborhood would be a great place to get a perspective on what the aging population was doing and thinking. So I turned my attention to two perfect examples:

— My neighbor Vi just turned 90, and she's a kick. Even though she had her left leg amputated two years ago because of a blood-clotting issue (not from diabetes), she has a spirit that just won't quit. Other people in her position would simply give up and die, but not Vi. Her doctors are amazed by how well she walks with her prosthetic leg, and she's always game to try new things. If I knock on her door and she's not home, chances are she's out on the ocean walk, or she's buzzing down to the village in her motorized wheelchair to do some shopping or go to the bank.

Although many of Vi's longtime friends have either died or gone to nursing homes, she has a great family and lots of young pals. She entertains often, and everyone wants to talk to her at a party. Vi's also always "dressed": You'll never find her in a tattered housecoat; rather, she'll greet you at the door in a fresh shirt, culottes or pressed pants, and a gold necklace and earrings. "You never know who you're going to meet," she says, so she's ready, no matter who comes calling.

What's Vi's secret? "I've always been interested in people," she told me. And she claims that taking hormones for more than 20 years has kept her memory sharp and her zest alive. She confided, "If I'm out of my hormones for a few days, I notice the difference. I'm not as sharp, I get into a slump, and I can feel a bit disoriented."

When I get to 90, I'd like to be like Vi—but I'd like to have both my legs!

— While 86-year-old Dorothy *does* have both of her legs, she also has half of her faculties. She shuffles around with her head down and a dour look on her face, and she has very few friends. I'm sure that even her family members who visit find it a chore, since she seems to have lost the will to live. She tends to only want to discuss her ailments, such as arthritis, bladder problems, and the first stages of Alzheimer's disease.

I look at Dorothy's groceries as she carries them back from the store in her walker and note that it's nothing healthy—cookies, candy, and alcohol. "Give up my bread, my pasta, and all my baked goods?" she asked in wonderment. "You must be joking! Why, I couldn't live without my goodies." Even though living with her "goodies" has only brought Dorothy 50 pounds of extra weight, mobility problems, and pain, she refuses to even consider parting with them. This woman is addicted to substances that she hopes will dull the edge of her trials yet are only doing the opposite . . . what a shame.

While these stories represent only two of the many faces of getting older, I hope you can see that it's possible to fully enjoy life as long as you're on this planet, rather than deciding that because you've reached a certain age, it's time to count down to death.

Looking for Answers

In taking a look at your own body, you may want to know more about what happens to it as the years progress. But where do you start? There are many books on the subject; and supplements, bioidentical hormones, cosmetic procedures, retirement communities, and life-extension programs abound. You may be baffled and overwhelmed by the array of material being presented, and I certainly understand how you feel. In these pages, I'll be giving you a fresh perspective, digging a little deeper beyond simply telling you to take a handful of vitamins.

I know from my work as a medical intuitive that there are certain components that can turn around chronic, degenerative disease and flood energy back into the body. So in order to be proactive about vibrant aging, understand that there are three main reasons for body breakdown: (1) addictions, (2) toxins, and (3) allergens.

As a medical intuitive, these three "agers" are very easy to see and are a big part of why people experience cancer, dementia, memory loss, arthritis, hearing loss, bladder problems, mobility concerns, decreasing skin elasticity, anxiety, depression, osteoporosis, balance issues, weakness, and vision problems—not to mention ending up in nursing homes. Addictions, toxins, and allergens all point to one problem: the slow, cell-by-cell demise of the human body. It's the death process.

In the next chapter, I'll discuss the effect of the "big three" on physical, emotional, and spiritual levels; and I'll give you some hints on how to release them from your life. When this is accomplished, you'll feel liberated, thus freeing your body to repair and regenerate.

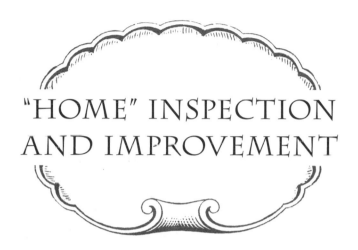

CHAPTER 2

"HOME" INSPECTION AND IMPROVEMENT

In this book, I want to help you easily navigate your way through your time on Earth, so I've given you some simple and practical strategies and tools to make your life a fun adventure. As you turn back the aging clock, it's important that you look at your body just as you would a house. This home of yours may be a little tired, worn out in spots, or in need of some shoring up here and there, but its beauty can absolutely be resurrected— it's just going to take a bit of elbow grease.

The Five Layers of Vibrant Aging

Let's get out our toolbox and get to work, remembering that there are many levels to being healthy while we age. When we become proactive about the physical layers of our home, then its emotional and spiritual ones will reveal themselves as well.

So with this in mind, I'd like to introduce you to the five layers of vibrant aging. Here, I'll give you a taste of how we're going to build on each of these elements as the book progresses so that we're optimally healthy, both inside and out.

1. The Appearance: How Things Look

- **Skin:** the walls of our house; the covering; our outer shell; what is apparent. In this regard, we're more than we appear to be.

- **Hair:** the roof of our house; our halo, our crown; our connection to the Divine. Let's wear our crown and connect to our higher power.

- **Eyes:** the windows of our home; the visionary; the seer. We choose to view the world with new eyes.

- **Ears:** listening to the still, small voice within. This is the voice of inner guidance.

Something to think about: We are more than we appear to be. How can we enhance and even change our physical appearance and our core energy so that we retain our youth and vitality?

2. The Structure: What Supports Us

- **Joints:** where the walls and floors of our house come together; flexibility; moving forward. Here we bend to the higher will.

- **Muscles:** the stairs of our home; the workers and load carriers. We lighten our burdens and ease our tensions.

- **Bones:** the structure and framework of our house; building; footing. We rebuild a firm foundation.

Something to think about: Where is our physical and emotional support? Are we supporting ourselves with positive thoughts and actions? How can we maintain a pain-free structure for the rest of our lives?

3. The Supply Lines: What Circulates Within Us

- **Blood:** those who live in our house; the life force; the river. We flow with the vitality of life. We rebuild our cells with our high-quality blood.

- **Heart:** the pulse; the kitchen and living space of our house; love; forgiveness; acceptance. We accept that change is inevitable, and we accept others. We take care of our heart.

- **Lungs:** the good, clean air of our home; the Divine healing breath within our body. It's easy to breathe deeply.

- **Stomach:** the furnace of our house; fuel, power; digestion. We easily digest life's experiences.

- **Pancreas:** sweetness in life. We look beyond our desire for "goodies" that overtax our pancreas to activities and people that give us the "sweet" life.

Something to think about: How can we provide our major organs and systems with the healthiest foods and supplements so that they support us and give us cell-building materials? What are our beliefs about unlimited supply in our lives?

4. The Waste Systems: How We Detoxify

- **Colon:** the plumbing; the pipes; the sanitation system. We don't want to hold on to old stuff.

- **Lymph:** the waste system that runs beneath the skin. We release the past and keep moving forward.

- **Kidneys:** flushing out impurities in the body. We keep bodily fluids, minerals, and electrolytes in balance.

- **Bladder:** the waterworks; fluidity; liquidity. We keep the liquids flowing to remove toxins and not get caught up in emotions.

Something to think about: We deeply trust that the universe is bringing us everything we need. We realize that we no longer need to hang on to outmoded beliefs and past issues. We feed our bodies nourishing foods that keep us clean, detoxified, and healthy.

5. Energy and Creativity: What Excites Us

- **Genitals:** sex; gender; passion; creativity. We give our whole self to life, which becomes our lover.

- **Energy:** the buzz of happy, life-giving power in our house; steam; drive; fuel. We aim to keep this high, sustainable, and clean-burning energy.

- **Aura:** emanation; field of manifestation. We put out, and draw to ourselves, a wonderful quality of life.

- **Brain:** the work center of our home; genius; creativity; intuition. We have a sharp mind.

- **Memory:** the database of our house; the bank; the repository. We remember everything. Our mind and memory are sharp and clear.

- **Spirit:** our essence, aliveness, vitality, and individuality. This connection to the Divine is what we leave on the planet after our earthly time is over.

Something to think about: We want to give our whole spirit to life and not hold back. We know that our time on Earth is short and very precious. We are one with the Divine, and we emanate this Divine presence wherever we go.

Protecting Your House

The key to healthy aging is not just a matter of addition, but rather one of subtraction. You must simply remove what weakens and add what strengthens.

Now I'd like to go through each part of the body and stress how addictions, toxins, and allergens have an effect on your overall health, and show you how you can protect your home from their ravaging effects.

Skin

The skin represents the walls of your house. It's your covering, the way you appear, or that which is apparent. On the physical level, many things can damage the skin:

- An addiction to a substance such as **sugar** breaks down skin cells and ages them more quickly. Rebuild cells by keeping sugars low. And stay out of "the cancer zone" by eliminating sugar from your diet altogether, because cancer cells need glucose to divide and proliferate.

- If frequently consumed, a toxin like **coffee** can age and wrinkle the skin, since it pulls the water right out of it. I can almost always spot a coffee drinker right away: He or she will have wrinkled, orange skin and emanate a toxic vibration.

- **Sun damage** contributes to premature aging. Of course sun worshipping is very seductive (who doesn't want that glow?), but it comes at quite a price.

- As we age, **bruising** can be a problem, as small, broken capillaries show up on the hands, feet, and legs. I grew up in the '60s, when beehive hairdos and tight skirts and sweaters were all the rage. So were panty girdles—I wore one all through high school, and as a result, I have several spider veins on my thighs. Sometimes on a Sunday morning when I notice that my husband is reading *The New York Times* and crossing his legs (not a good thing to be doing for vein health), he'll look over his glasses, smile, and tell me that he's cultivating his varicosities.

  Bruising and broken veins point to a circulation problem, as they're indicating that cell walls may be weakening. Rutin, a bioflavonoid, is a buckwheat supplement that can

help repair broken capillaries; it's available at
health-food stores.

- **Stress** can age the skin—worry or anxiety
  can actually add years to how you look. You
  can't always eliminate stress, but you *can* create strategies so that the pressure in your life
  doesn't take you down. There are many ways
  to relieve stress so that you're not containing
  or holding on to it: Take a break, get a massage, go for a walk, meditate, make love to
  your significant other, or do anything that
  relaxes you.

Take a look at your skin and appreciate it. Later on in
the book, I'll give you suggestions for supplements that
you can take to strengthen and repair it, but for now,
just breathe love and gratitude into your skin—as it is
right now.

Hair

Toxins in the body will manifest as thinning, dull,
lifeless tresses that are dry, brittle, and break off easily.
You can get great hair by drinking water, using high-
quality fats and oils in your diet, balancing your thyroid
gland, and working on digestion.

Yet your hair is also your crown, your halo or aura—
your connection to the Divine. How connected to God
do you feel? You must wear your crown, build your self-
esteem, and be proud . . . all of which will contribute to
thick, healthy, shiny hair.

Eyes

Eyes are the windows of your home, and they represent your interior and exterior vision.

How can you get great vision? By removing toxins and poisons, cleaning up your liver (which sweeps toxins out of the blood), and supplementing yourself with nourishing food and vitamins. Rest and adequate sleep revitalizes the eyes; later on, I'll also give you a set of exercises and a unique tool that will help you strengthen them.

Now let's take a look at the deeper meaning of the eyes, which correlate to one of the body's power-healing energy centers. As soon as you get in touch with your soul or spiritual aspect, you'll radiate love to everyone you meet through your eyes—which will then become bathed in liquid light and take on an obvious luminescence.

In addition, the eyes represent your own view of yourself. If you're having physical problems in this area, perhaps you need to take the time to reexamine your vision for your life. Where are you going? What are your goals—can you see them?

Ears

Are you listening to your still, small voice within? Can you hear your inner guidance? Is there someone in your life whom you don't want to listen to, perhaps your critical parent or spouse? Is this the voice of your boss, which you'd really like to turn off?

If your ears feel crackly or full, this is usually a sign of fungus in your ears. It can also be the hallmark of an allergy to yeasts, molds, or dairy products. (I offer many suggestions to help with such allergies later in the book.)

Joints

Joints represent the flexibility in your bodily home and can be improved by removing certain foods from your diet. Did you know that wheat products can cause inflammation, arthritis, and joint pain? Take a temporary break from consuming wheat products and substitute other grains such as rice, 100 percent rye, or quinoa, which don't cause inflammation and pain.

Recently, I met a woman at a spa who was in her 70s but looked marvelous and healthy to me. However, as we sat down to dinner, she broke into her bread roll, and I could see that her hands were gnarled and twisted with arthritis. I suggested that she stop eating any wheat-based products, and these days her hands feel great.

One of the body's great miracles is that it knows what it wants—so when that's what you provide, it will repair itself.

Now let's look at the joints in terms of flexibility and being open to new ideas. Are you flexible in your approach? Are you open to suggestions? Are you moving forward? Are you bending to the higher will? How you answer these questions will give you great insight into the state of your joint health.

Muscles

Muscles are the workers and load carriers in your house. Did you know that they can feel much more free and flexible when you improve digestion? Toxins in the system tighten muscles, but good digestion improves the quality of nutrition supplied to *all* parts of your body. Muscles and joints also respond to stretching exercise, as lengthening and strengthening your body will help keep you flexible and pain free.

Let's look at muscles on a higher level. Are you carrying too heavy a load? Are you encumbered by financial strain? Are you caring for children or elderly parents or otherwise working full-time? Is your burden weakening your body? Take a look—maybe it's time to make some changes and lighten the load. Let someone else do the work.

Bones

Bones, the structure of your home, are built by the hormones estrogen and progesterone. Estrogen breaks down bones, while progesterone builds them back up—so in order to have strong and healthy bones, you need to take a careful, proactive look at hormone balancing. Yes, you need good nutrition and supplementation, but calcium may not be enough as you age, no matter how beneficial it is. Hormones are a key factor here.

Bones and structure also represent your belief system. What you believe in and what you stand for make up your strength and foundation; thus, doing the inner work of believing in yourself will strengthen your very bones.

Heart

The heart is the life and pulse center of your home. How can you help your heart as you get older? Again, subtracting toxins, addictions, and allergens is a great start.

Did you know that just the simple step of removing stimulants from your diet will regulate your heart rate, or that red meat supports its electrical firing? What about the fact that excessive consumption of sugar and starch can lay plaque down on your arteries and weaken your cell walls? The exciting news is that you can now make healthy dietary choices and take specific nutrients to dissolve that plaque.

On the inner level, examine your heart and discover any areas where you haven't forgiven a past issue or old wound. Working on your *emotional* heart is the highest level of personal self-mastery.

Lungs

Lungs represent the "breath of life" in our bodies. Did you know that the digestive system, sinuses, and lungs are all connected? Indeed, they're actually on the same acupuncture meridian. So when we clean up our guts, our lungs and sinuses will also improve.

Examine the quality of the air that you breathe—is it pure and clean? Maybe you need an air filter in your home. In addition, remember to take deep, full breaths of life, as deep breathing has been shown to be a positive factor in vibrant aging.

Stomach

The stomach is the gut and the power center of our bodily home, so here we need to look at the management of power.

Are you giving your power away—investing it in people, places, and things outside of yourself—or are you keeping much of it for your own use? If you have a strong level of personal power and self-esteem, you'll usually have better digestion on the physical level. Also, take a look at what and how you're eating. The rate at which you're digesting food and the use of digestive enzymes can improve the quality of your inner furnace.

Colon

The colon is the waste system of your house, so you'll want it to be working optimally. A daily bowel movement keeps toxins to a minimum, but having a decent one every day can be a great quest. It depends on avoiding foods to which you might be allergic, notably dairy products; eating plenty of roughage, such as fresh vegetables and fiber; drinking lots of water; making sure that there's adequate magnesium in your diet; and balancing your thyroid gland.

Emotionally, getting rid of old garbage in your thoughts by not hanging on to fear and worry is a big factor here. Letting go and letting God—that is, just flowing with life—relates to this part of your body.

Kidneys

The kidneys are located in the middle of your back, on either side of your spine. They're major detoxification organs that filter out fluid from the blood and convert it into urine, which is expelled through the bladder. Kidneys clean unwanted substances and protect the blood from lethal conditions such as hypertension, coronary artery disease, and congestive heart failure. Consistently high blood pressure can damage these organs, and heavy-metal toxicity can lead to kidney disease.

As part of the aging process, the kidneys diminish in size: Studies show that those of an 80-year-old have shrunk by 20 percent, thus decreasing filtering function. In order to remove toxins, keep drinking water, especially in hot weather. Drinking plenty of water also prevents kidney stones, which can be produced thanks to too much caffeine, alcohol, and chemicals. And it greatly helps your kidneys if you release the past emotionally.

Bladder

The bladder is a pouch that holds a specific amount of urine, until it receives the impulse that tells you it's time to void. The bladder represents washing away all the toxins and poisons that you accumulate during the day from the foods you eat and the chemicals you expose yourself to. You flush out anything that isn't useful or helpful, and you fill yourself up with the new. Therefore, it's very important to work on releasing your anger and fear.

Water, and lots of it, is fundamental to refreshing and vitalizing your kidneys and bladder. In addition, sugar consumption can aggravate bladder bacteria—thus creating urgency and frequency—so take in minimal amounts. Acidifying the urine with vitamin C or unsweetened cranberry juice can be a useful strategy, as is taking herbs such as juniper, buchu, and marshmallow root. If you're a woman, you may also need low-dose estrogen cream applied vaginally to strengthen tissue at the neck of the urethra.

Liver

The liver is a digestive, excretory, and endocrine organ. It secretes bile salts for fat digestion; stores vitamins and minerals; synthesizes blood-clotting factors; and is involved in the regulation of carbohydrates, fats, and proteins. Excess cholesterol is excreted through the liver via bile. It also makes urea, metabolizes alcohol, and helps with the detoxification of drugs and other foreign substances.

Use milk thistle or other herbs to detoxify your liver, and remove known toxins from your diet. Continue to support and detoxify this organ if you're taking prescription medication. As the liver represents anger in Chinese medicine, work on related issues.

Gallbladder

The gallbladder is a small, pear-shaped sac that stores bile and is involved in the breakdown of fats in the diet. Gallstones form because of poor fat digestion; over time they can increase in size and number, to the point that they clog the bile ducts and prevent the liver from producing bile. Gallbladder removal is a very common surgical procedure—in fact, it accounts for more than 500,000 surgeries each year in the United States alone. Add more vegetables and fiber to your diet. Change your oils from saturated and trans fats to olive, nut, or seed oils. Take bile salts to help your ducts function properly. And on an energetic level, the gallbladder represents richness in life, so open up to and accept the riches of your kingdom.

Genitals

The genitals represent the "beat": passion, sexuality, gender, connection to the planet, and vulnerability. If we balance our hormones and have great energy, then we're ready to experience great sex. In the normal aging process, hormone levels decline, thus sending libido out the window. Fortunately, thanks to the growing interest in bioidentical hormone balancing in the last few years, engaging in pleasurable sexual activity is now something we can continue to enjoy throughout our lives—it's not relegated to the younger generation. Caring, treasuring, and nurturing intimacy only gets better with age.

Blood

Blood represents the life force, and it depends on exercise, oxygenation, and removing (or at least decreasing) toxins and addictions. Blood is the river and flow of existence: Are you flowing with what it's offering, or are you stuck? Are there boulders and rocks in your river?

On another level, blood represents passion and enthusiasm for life. When I see people, I can immediately tell the quality of their life force—their level of will to live. Check inside and ask yourself how passionate and enthusiastic *you* are about things and the direction you're going. Find out what's holding you back from experiencing true passion in your life.

Brain

The brain is the repository of all thoughts and memories, so how can we nourish it? Strange as it may seem, we do so through our guts. Nutrition from our stomach enters the bloodstream through the digestive tract wall; consequently, a diet that's full of sugar and chemicals won't support the brain. Over time, these toxic culprits, as well as pollutants from the environment, cause our brain cells to atrophy, wither, and die. But as soon as we clean up the neurotoxins, our brain cells regenerate again. For example, when I wasn't even 40 years old, I lost my memory and couldn't think straight. Yet when I cleaned up my diet, my brain cells regenerated, and I got my memory back right away.

Another factor in brain function is hormones, so if your memory is declining, take heart! You're not necessarily developing Alzheimer's disease—you may just require some estrogen or testosterone. You merely need to do some body balancing so that your body can regenerate and repair. You can also keep your brain active by writing your life story.

Energy

This is our steam, drive, desire, and fuel. Energy should be an eternal fountain that comes from within, available to us like a vast storehouse that pours into, and out of, us at any time. Unfortunately, this is often not the case—I see so many people who are tired, listless, dull, and lacking vital energy.

The answer here is simple: Do your best to take energy-draining substances out of your diet, and remove energy-draining people from your life. I teach people that addictive substances (such as junk food, sugar, soft drinks, and alcohol) run away from our bodies and take all of our life energy with them. Human beings can be the same way, too, so who in your life is dragging you down? Try to surround yourself with positive, supportive individuals who believe in you and your goals. In addition, find out what you love to do, and then set about doing it.

Aura

The aura or electromagnetic field represents our glow or magnetism. In Renaissance paintings, people were often depicted with glowing halos over their heads— these were spiritual masters, saints, and sages who emanated Divine love. We can also have this vibrant glow, which is visible to the trained eye.

How can you increase the width of your electromagnetic field? Well, when you remove the "usual suspects" of toxins, addictions, and allergens, this automatically affects that field, changes your energy, and causes you to become more attractive. As a result, you become more connected spiritually and send out a loving vibration, thus drawing in all of the experiences and people you want to have into your life. You become the magnet that pulls the things you desire to you.

In summary, in order to take care of all of the parts of your house I've listed in this chapter, you must remove as many toxic substances as you can from your body; supplement, love, and support yourself; and give your body a chance to regenerate and repair. It will do so—I've seen it happen in men and women of *all* ages.

Let's take a closer look at addictions and how they can be overcome.

CHAPTER 3

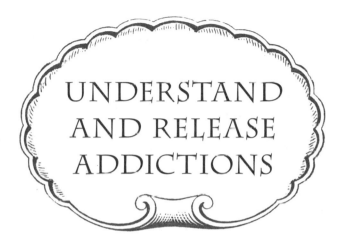

UNDERSTAND
AND RELEASE
ADDICTIONS

• •

If you're sick, chances are you're addicted to certain foods, behaviors, and thoughts. Anything that has power over you and that you have difficulty letting go of is an addiction. For example, dwelling on the past can be just as damaging as being hooked on coffee, alcohol, or chocolate, because it holds you back in life.

In fact, noted physician and author Deepak Chopra claims that all illness is the result of addiction. I couldn't agree more—this has been my observation for the past 25 years. In fact, when I used to work as an allergy-testing technician, I noted that as soon as people removed the substances they were addicted to, all their symptoms miraculously went away.

This is why Dr. Doris Rapp, a well-known expert in environmental medicine, suggests that patients replace everything they currently consume with things they don't normally eat for five days. She's noticed over and over again that chronic complaints disappear and health improves when this happens. (Please visit: **www.drrapp. com**.)

In my work as a medical intuitive, almost everyone I see has an addiction of some sort. I can tell that something is hooked into them, be it physical or emotional, and it's robbing their vital force and taking them down cell by cell. I might see gray or black around them—a dark or negative force that's stealing their precious stamina and vitality. Something has a hold on them, and I know that they're addicted.

From this deep spiritual perspective, I believe that we should all be free: No particular substance, person, place, or physical possession should have us in its clutches. I call this "the climb." Now, many of us are content to go around and around the bottom of a mountain, but very few want to do the work to ascend it. Just as in real mountaineering, the trek I'm proposing will require concentration and discipline.

As we age, we'll do a lot better if we're prepared, focused, and free of excess baggage, including anything that's a toxin, allergen, or poison. The mountain that we are, will be stronger and more supportive as we age if we're willing to examine our issues and give up the items we're addicted to.

The aging game is not to be taken lightly. In order to stave off the ravages of old age, we've got to get busy and become prepared—now!

Climbing Out of the Addictive Process

We're spiritual beings—our entire raison d'être is to operate from a conscious perspective. We're here to make a difference on this planet, and as soon as we turn the corner of age 50, this becomes all the more apparent. So the emission of radiant, clear, positive energy from our physical bodies is very significant in relationship to our manifestation ability.

Your aura or electromagnetic field is what you use to draw people, things, and experiences into your life. As you desire to manifest or attract the best to you on a material and spiritual level, an emanation of glowing energy is essential, and it can only come from having a clear and detoxified physical body. Addictions cloud your aura, and even a simple doughnut or cup of coffee can muddy your field. Try it sometime by ingesting your favorite "poison" and waiting 20 minutes. You'll quickly see that the result is a tired, worn-out body that's temporarily removed or disengaged from life.

The ability to effectively manifest is in direct proportion to how clear your aura is. So if you want to make the climb out of addiction, take out a sheet of paper and a pen and follow these steps:

1. Make a list of all the **things** you're hooked on. These can be foods (such as candy, bread, or chocolate), beverages (such as soda, coffee, or milk), or chemicals (including drugs and alcohol).

2. Next, make a list of everything that might be an addictive **behavior,** such as staying up late, working too hard, worrying too much, overspending, overeating,

nagging at your partner, remaining in an unsatisfying job or relationship, being a pack rat, or the like.

3. Finally, make a list of any **thoughts** that have you in their vise grip. These are what you find yourself thinking about most often, including dwelling on the past, self-deprecating beliefs (such as *I'm not good enough, I'm not worthy, I'm not intelligent,* or *There is never enough*), and so forth.

Of course no one wants to be mired in negativity. Thankfully, author Eve Brinton shares a simple and practical technique for switching out of negative thoughts in her book *Instant Happiness with the Energy Exchange* (available through **www.evebrinton.com**).

Brinton believes that changing habitual negative thoughts and reframing them into positive ones can be accomplished in less than a minute. To that end, think of something positive right now: Maybe it was when you flew over the Grand Canyon in a helicopter; or when you were in your grandmother's garden, feeling peace and happiness wash over you. As soon as you find yourself dwelling in negativity, find that positive image and draw it into your consciousness. You'll instantly notice the difference.

As the Dalai Lama teaches, why should you allow anyone to disturb the freedom of your thoughts? Your material possessions can be taken from you, but your thoughts remain your own. And because *you* create your thoughts, they can't have any power over you. Thanks to Brinton's Energy Exchange, you can master your mental activity and be free.

The Law of Attraction

As you climb your own mountain on the journey of personal self-mastery, your desire is to be as free as a bird so that you can be moved by the universe and go wherever your soul wants you to. Remember what I learned from my near-death experience . . . since life is short and so precious, use the law of attraction to draw good into your life.

As a medical intuitive, I see subtle energies: For example, coffee carries the emanation of anger and irritation; and the energy of excessive alcohol use is like a "zing," taking away the body's life force like a feather in the wind. The moment you consume a substance like coffee, you put its vibration into your field. Then, because like attracts like, you'll probably pull angry and irritating experiences to you such as losing your car keys, getting involved in minor altercations, or blowing things out of proportion.

How can you tell if a food or beverage is really affecting you? That's easy—take your pulse. An easy-to-find pulse point can be found on the carotid artery that supplies blood to your brain, which is located on either side of your neck just below your jaw. Find that point, become familiar with what your normal pulse rate feels like, and then start testing. Twenty minutes after you've had a cup of coffee (or consumed anything that you're concerned about), test your pulse again: If it's elevated or racing, this is an obvious sign that your body is rebelling against the poison or toxin you've ingested.

Pulse testing is one of the ways in which traditional allergists determine potential sensitivities, but you already know the answer intuitively. I'm always amazed when people tell me during a reading that they're aware that coffee, cola, corn, sugar, and other stimulants affect them—yet they can't believe how calm and happy they feel when they give them up.

Coffee also clouds the aura, hardens the prostate gland, causes jitters and an irregular heartbeat, pulls fluids out of the body, blocks the lymphatic system, contributes to cellulite, and a dozen other effects. So the easy and obvious answer is to switch to decaf for a few weeks. A good decaffeinated roast has the same taste and smell as real coffee, but it doesn't have the kick. Decaf might not have any deleterious effects, but by consuming it, you're still keeping the memory, taste, essence, and vibration of coffee alive.

Remember that you're climbing the mountain, so the next step is to eliminate the decaffeinated java and switch to herbal or green tea (make sure it has low amounts of caffeine). You're not giving coffee up just to give it up—you're releasing this addiction, and others, to lengthen your life. I know that there are studies that indicate coffee is beneficial. But in my opinion, these studies don't show the drink's effects on one's aura, heart, or genitals . . . or, indeed, one's *life*.

The same goes for sugar, which may taste ever so good to you. But what does it do to your energy, your nervous system, your precious pancreas, and your cell walls? Sweetness should come from life, so this is where following your dreams and living your passion take priority. When you're happy and fulfilled in your work and play, you really won't be interested in sweets.

It Comes with a Gift

Keep in mind that your willingness to set aside addictions always comes with a gift. I believe that we're all being watched over by angels and towering beings at all times who are shepherding us and guiding us.

As soon as we give up an addictive behavior, the next step will be revealed. Just watch the phone ring, a job opportunity arise, a pure white feather land in our lap, or a serendipitous benefit appear seemingly out of nowhere. One door closes on what's no longer healthy, but another one opens to something better. This is confirmation that the universe knows that we are climbing the mountain and are willing to give up what no longer serves us in favor of what *will* benefit us (and humankind). Then the addiction is no longer viewed with seduction but with recognition of what it can—and will—do to our precious life force and cellular tissue. We make the decision to leave it behind and attract something priceless.

I've personally benefited from vibrant health for the past 25 years because I gave up coffee, wine, chocolate-chip cookies (by the dozen), homemade bread, and lots of cheese. I got my life back, and there has never been a moment where I thought the choice wasn't worth it. The smell of coffee and the taste of chocolate simply aren't appealing to me anymore. My addictions have turned into passions: I'm passionate about teaching, I'm passionate about communicating, and I'm passionate about health. It's as if the angels have given me a mandate to empower *you* to get healthy, too, so that you'll be able to complete your destiny as I have.

Sure, I have the occasional stray into "no-no land." I'll have a glass of wine or a sweet dessert on occasion, but it better be good. My husband and I might share a crème brûlée on our anniversary, for instance, or I may enjoy a small slice of my daughter's wonderful pie at a family gathering. But I know that I'll be feeling and seeing the effects of those choices very soon. I might wake up feeling a little tired or grouchy; my eyes might be puffy, and my clothes might be tight; or, on the rare occasions I have bread or pasta, my hands will become stiff. After three days of eating bread, my arthritis will return, so it's really not worth it for me. I'm climbing the mountain, and these so-called temptations simply don't entice me anymore.

Addictions and Medications

What about people who are addicted to medication? After all, every prescription drug has side effects. Yet you'd be surprised by the number of folks who are on medication and would rather have the side effects than change their habits or research alternatives. If they would just give up their habit, their symptoms would back off, but these people choose to stay addicted.

For example, at age 62, Gretchen had bladder problems and was hooked on sweets and alcohol. Sure, she had reason to be addicted to these items: She had a 28-year-old son who was running amok—he was stealing money from her, had quit his job, and was draining her dry and disrespecting her. She felt powerless to stand up for herself and reclaim her own life, so she soothed her wounds with red wine and pound cake. Bacteria had built up in her body, probably due to a lack of hydration, so she was put on diuretics and sulfa drugs to take care of it.

She's now faced with bladder surgery, rounds of antibiotics, and a compounded set of medical concerns that will probably set her on a careening course to premature aging. Will she change? I hope so, but many people like Gretchen are addicted to the drama of their emotional lives. This keeps them in the fury of the hurricane, which is familiar territory. Rather than make some simple lifestyle changes, it's easier for such men and women to stay stuck and medicated.

Now I'm a firm believer in traditional Western medicine *when it is needed*. I know that drugs can save lives because I grew up in a medical household: My mother was a dietitian, and both my father and grandfather were medical doctors. In our house, the physician was God. Today, things are different. I know that each of us can be God and the doctor ourselves, and other practitioners form our own healing team.

Let's remember this basic concept: *The body knows how to get well.* But optimal health takes a deeper level of commitment than some people are willing to make. Because you're reading this book, I know that you're willing to point your compass toward aging optimally, beautifully, and vibrantly.

In the next chapter, we'll see what kind of impact environmental toxins have on us.

CHAPTER 4

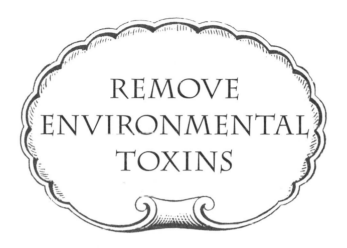

REMOVE
ENVIRONMENTAL
TOXINS

· ·

If you're in your 50s or 60s as I am, you know that we were born in a different era—it was safe to walk to school, our mothers made all our meals from scratch, there was much less pollution, our food wasn't loaded with chemicals, and life wasn't as stressful.

However, we also grew up routinely being exposed to coal, lead, and cigarette smoke. I remember chewing the lead paint off the side rail of my bed when I was a little girl, for instance, and it tasted bitter and acrid. My parents smoked when my siblings and I were small children, and we had a coal-burning furnace that my older brother stoked every morning. My sister and I would shiver on the metal grate above the furnace while we waited for it to crank up, and as we danced out of our pajamas and into our underpants, of course we breathed in plenty of smoky, coal-fire fumes. It's no wonder that my weak link is my lungs.

Given our histories and the amount of toxins we've ingested over the years, most of us will find that it's high time to detoxify ourselves. In this chapter, I'll show you how to do just that by focusing on the liver, the gallbladder, the kidneys, the bladder, and the digestive system.

The Liver

As a digestive, excretory, and endocrine organ, the liver sweeps and filters the blood and synthesizes blood-clotting factors. It stores vitamins and minerals—and toxins and poisons—and is involved in the regulation of carbohydrates, fats, and proteins, as well as hormone production. Cholesterol is manufactured in the liver, and excess amounts are excreted through it via bile. (Urea is another by-product made here.) Detoxification of drugs and other foreign substances takes place through the liver, which is why its function is carefully evaluated before prescribing medication that could overtax it. Alcohol is metabolized through the liver, so excessive consumption can severely damage this organ.

The liver is located under the rib cage, just underneath the right breast. You can find it by counting up two to three ribs from your bottom rib and placing your fingers about three inches below your right nipple. Now this could be interesting, depending upon where your nipple is located—at age 70, it might be a little lower than at age 50! Nevertheless, if you press on this area and it feels sore, your liver is probably toxic.

If you're worried about your liver, a close look at the toxins you're ingesting will help you make better choices. Along with following a healthy diet and doing your best to keep poisons out of the equation, you can take some liver-detoxification herbs or green drinks and fresh-vegetable juices. Try raw or lightly steamed fennel, which is a delicious herb that tastes like licorice *and* detoxifies your liver, too.

Your health-food store will be able to recommend the best herbs to help you here—the most common one is milk thistle, which has been known to assist in liver support as well as detoxification. The dose is usually one capsule with breakfast and dinner for about two months; then take up to four months off and repeat for another two months. Note that when you start taking liver herbs, you'll notice that your bowel movements will be very smelly for the first few days . . . whew! That's okay, though, because it's a sign of detoxification.

Indeed, there are numerous benefits resulting from detoxifying your liver. For example, you'll notice that your eyesight improves. Here's how this happens: Blood circulates throughout the body and supplies nutrients to your cells, including those of your skin, hair, fingernails, and eyes. When you clean your liver, you have better-quality blood circulating throughout your system, so your vision will improve. Try it for a while—I'll bet that when you remove toxic substances from your diet, you won't be reaching for your glasses as often. At your next examination, your eye doctor might even say that your sight has improved or that your vision hasn't declined as much as it should have for your age.

There are also liver points in the hands and feet, which can be found midway between your thumbs and first fingers in the fleshy part of the hands, and just behind the fleshy pads in the front balls of the feet.

Although you might find these points to be tender, go ahead and gently massage them twice a day.

This vital part of your body is termed "the seat of anger" in Chinese medicine, so during liver detoxification, know that it's common for anger issues to rise to the surface. It would be a good idea to take this opportunity to deal with such issues once and for all, and finally release them from your body.

When I think about the importance of the liver, I'm reminded of my friends Bonnie and John, who have been pursuing a wellness path for the past 25 years. At age 84, John does daily stretching exercises and plays golf, and he's actively involved in business and investments. Bonnie plays golf or tennis every day—not bad for 81 years of age. Since her locker was once next to mine at the tennis club, over the years we've shared many avenues to optimal health with each other. This couple takes specific supplements and eats a healthy diet, avoiding offending foods. Neither of them is on any medication, but Bonnie does take natural hormones.

I'm proud to see both John and Bonnie doing so well—in my opinion, they're the healthiest people I know. They look about 20 years younger than they really are, probably because they're out there having fun, while many of their counterparts are either dead or "old crocks."

Liver detoxification is one of the elements that my friends focus on. They only eat organic food; they don't have coffee in their home; their alcohol intake is minimal; they stick to eating healthy fats, which they keep low; and from time to time, they go on a liver-detoxification program.

What can *you* do to improve your liver function? Number one: Release your addictions to coffee, alcohol, chocolate, cigarettes, and recreational or prescription drugs. If you do ingest these items, seek out a Chinese acupuncturist for specially made herbal formulas to detoxify your liver and improve the quality of your blood.

The Gallbladder

Why do so many individuals need to have their gallbladders removed? Well, many people are addicted to eating large quantities of nuts for snacks, and high-protein and high-fat diets can be a real burden on the gallbladder, which is responsible for fat handling. Over time, fatty deposits collect here, and it can become difficult to digest fats—leading to the creation of gallstones, pain, nausea, or a full-blown gallbladder attack.

Two years ago, I had just such an attack three days before I was to lead a trip to Tuscany, Italy. This was not fun. I turned pea green, existed on chicken broth and steamed vegetables, and eschewed fat of all kinds until things calmed down. When I returned home, I did a gallbladder flush to expel the fatty deposits, and I felt so much better.

I don't recommend that you do a gallbladder flush unless you're monitored by a health professional. If the flush isn't done correctly, it could lead to a fatty deposit getting stuck in a bile duct, which may be an emergency situation. But if you suspect that you have a fatty gallbladder, there are many protocols for flushes that you can explore with your health-care provider.

The Kidneys

My client Len had quite a shocking and painful experience when he returned from working on an AIDS project in Africa. After having been in Sudan for three months, traveling out into the field giving presentations on AIDS prevention for local people, he developed kidney stones. Len realized that the lack of potable water in the region was a huge factor in limiting his intake, so he hadn't been hydrating himself sufficiently. Fortunately for him, there's a relatively new ultrasound procedure that's designed to break up kidney stones, disintegrating them so that they can be passed less painfully.

Yes, in a hot part of the world like Africa, it's imperative to drink water because it flushes impurities out of the kidneys. But this isn't just an issue for Africans—here in the West, over and over we see elderly people with kidney and bladder issues because they don't drink enough water. It turns out that they're afraid of having to go to the bathroom too often. Less water equals fewer pee-pee breaks; more water equals more pee-pee breaks, but it also results in fewer kidney and bladder problems.

Taking care of your kidneys by cutting down on coffee and alcohol and increasing your water intake can be an important step in detoxification. There are also various kidney cleanses available through your health-care practitioner or health-food store.

The Bladder

To pee or not to pee is the question on many post-menopausal women's minds. When we were younger, we could hold on for hours without emptying our bladders . . . now it's different. We go before we leave home, we go at our first appointment of the day, and we even have to go in the middle of the night! And men have urinary-tract problems, too—they could be suffering from an enlarged prostate gland, which presses on the urethra, thus affecting their urine flow or stream.

Sometimes bacteria builds up in the bladder, causing inflammation at the neck of the urethra. This narrows the top of the urinary tract where it connects to the bladder, so voiding is incomplete, leaving a few tablespoons of urine behind. Then the body's heat warms up this small amount of urine, along with the bacteria, thus causing the feeling of urgency or frequency. It can even lead to a full-blown bladder infection.

Here are some prevention strategies:

- Reduce sugar consumption, which then reduces bacteria formation.

- Drink more water.

- Drink two ounces of unsweetened cranberry juice two times a day.

- Take cranberry capsules or bladder herbs such as juniper or buchu.

- If you're a woman, see your doctor and get a prescription for estradiol or estriol cream. This can strengthen the urinary-tract wall and prevent bacteria from creeping up the urethra. Try Vagifem, a vaginal insert; or Estring, a vaginal ring—both of which contain a low dose of timed-release estrogen that can help strengthen tissue.

- Know that sexual intercourse, oral sex, and using a vibrator can irritate delicate urinary-tract tissue. Be sure to void immediately after having sex. Drink more water, use bladder herbs, and acidify the urine with high doses of vitamin C three times a day for a few days.

- Eradicate Candida yeast, which is a major cause of bladder issues.

- See your doctor if a bladder problem or infection persists beyond three days.

A Home Remedy for the Bladder

This remedy was given to me years ago by Dr. Jim Mac-Kimmie, author of *Presence of Angels: A Healer's Life* (Knowing Heart Press). Jim's a wonderful chiropractor and healer who's a font of old-time wisdom. The concoction below has saved my bacon on a number of occasions when I've been on the verge of getting a bladder infection. It may seem to be a very odd remedy, but it works like a charm, and onions do have well-known antibacterial properties.

Follow these steps:

- Take 4 jumbo (must be jumbo) yellow cooking onions and quarter them.

- Drop the onions into 2 quarts of briskly boiling water.

- Boil for 20 minutes or until they're soft.

- Discard the onions.

- Drink 3 cups of the juice immediately, and take the balance of the liquid throughout the day or the next day. The broth is naturally sweet and pleasant tasting.

On a higher level, bladders represent holding on to fear. Some would say it's about anger, and of course that's part of fear, but many times I find that when people are going through turbulent periods, they're on edge, frozen in fear. As this emotion can precipitate a bladder infection or problem, drinking plenty of fluids to keep urine flowing is very important.

The Digestive System

We can't really talk about detoxifying the body without taking bowel movements (BMs) into consideration. The intestinal tract is the human body's central command post or "mission control." Think about it: What you put into your body affects what comes out of it.

What goes into the gut affects the entire machine, and many people's machinery is blocked!

On the physical level, there is almost no other quest as important as the perfect bowel movement. I should know, since as a young child, I suffered from constipation. With a lot of effort, I'd produce what might be termed a "feeble attempt" at a BM about once a week. My father was a doctor, and my mother was a dietitian—go figure! When I was tested for food allergies years later, I discovered that milk and cheese had been making me constipated. As soon as I eliminated dairy products from my diet, the BMs appeared like clockwork.

Your desire is to produce a six- to nine-inch product in the toilet at least once a day. If you're having difficulty with this, find out the foods you're sensitive to and eliminate them for a brief period of time. Balance your lower intestinal flora with probiotics, which help with digestion, absorption, assimilation, and immunity.

How's your water intake? It should be around two quarts a day. Fiber and roughage may also need to be increased, and liver and gallbladder functions should be supported. If low magnesium is the culprit, take 250 mg at bedtime. (And many people swear by aloe-vera juice, often taking two ounces at bedtime.) In addition, hormones play a role here, as a low-functioning thyroid or a sluggish liver can contribute to constipation.

On an emotional level, constipation can represent difficulty in letting go of a past issue or releasing control over events in our lives. Those emotionally "anal retentive" types among us are just the kind of people who are likely to become physically anal retentive. Sometimes it's hard to think of letting go and allowing the universe to take care of things—but when we're "hanging on," we often block good things from happening.

The opposite of constipation is diarrhea. If a person has loose stools, he or she is less likely to be toxic but may not be adequately absorbing nutrition. Thus, he or she isn't rebuilding the body. That's what happened to Arnold, who was aging quickly even though he was only 53.

As a medical intuitive, I see levels of toxicity in the body, including four visible "casts" or shades to facial skin: (1) An orange brown tint can be a clear sign of a coffee drinker; (2) a dull gray shows me that the thyroid is low; (3) a grayish, putty color can indicate cancer or a precancerous condition; and (4) a dull brown denotes constipation. But when I looked at Arnold's body, I could see that he was almost completely depleted because he'd been eating too many raw foods and sprouted nuts. This plan may have been beneficial for him in the short term or when he was younger and more digestively robust, but at his current age, he needed a balance between raw and cooked foods. Digestive enzymes and the addition of consistent, small amounts of protein in his diet helped slow his BMs down. Now, because he's absorbing his nutrition better, Arnold's body is rebuilding.

If this man's situation sounds familiar to you, try eating fewer husky grains like corn, and you'll have more formed bowel movements. Lightly steam your vegetables, and go easy on the fresh fruit for a while—this could be the difference you're looking for. Again, taking digestive enzymes and using probiotics to balance lower-colon flora is effective.

Now take a close look at what you eat. Everything that you ingest has an effect on your intestinal tract and bowel movements. In the seven-day experiment I've suggested, when you set aside all the food items that are toxic or keeping you addicted, you'll probably notice significant improvements in your bowel movements.

A Word about Chemical Poisons

We're surrounded by a sea of chemicals, which is relatively new information. We once figured that plastics were pretty benign and user-friendly, for instance, but it turns out that not only do they clog our landfills, they also enter our food chain, our water supply, and our bodies. High levels of chemicals leached from plastics in a nearby landfill were found in a Canadian river not long ago—because these chemicals mimic estrogens, a percentage of the male fish were found to have female characteristics, and some female fish were found to have male as well as female characteristics.

According to a recent *USA Today* article that cited research in the publication *Reproductive Toxicology,* the level of bisphenol A—which is used in plastic baby bottles, dental sealants, and metal-can linings—exceeds current safety standards. This chemical has been shown to have hormonelike activity and has been linked to obesity, early puberty, hyperactivity, abnormal sexual behavior, and interrupted reproductive cycles.

It's scary to think how deeply these chemicals have penetrated our bodies and our environment. What kind of new generations of children are we raising?

As estrogens are produced in the liver, we should examine our food-storage methods. Xenoestrogens are estrogen-like substances that are found in dry-cleaning fluids, pesticides, and plastic materials. Look at all the food we purchase that's wrapped in plastic—then we get it home and store it in plastic film or bags. Worse still, we heat our food by wrapping it in plastic and putting it in the microwave, only to have these chemicals impregnate what we eat. Yikes!

As a result of the information that has come to light about estrogen-like substances, there are now many natural products available that can reduce estrogen levels in the body. Cruciferous vegetables, such as cabbage, kale, broccoli, cauliflower, brussels sprouts, and bok choy help detoxify estrogens. You can eat as much of these as you like, but you can also purchase them in capsule form and take one capsule with meals. Diindolylmethane (DIM) naturally occurs in cruciferous vegetables and is thought to have anticancer and antioxidant properties because it helps metabolize estrogen. Turmeric, a spice familiar in India and part of the curry family, can be useful in detoxifying estrogens—the dose is one capsule with breakfast and dinner.

Thanks to the information in this chapter, you're now well on your way to being detoxified. Next, let's take a close look at the role of allergens in the aging process.

CHAPTER 5

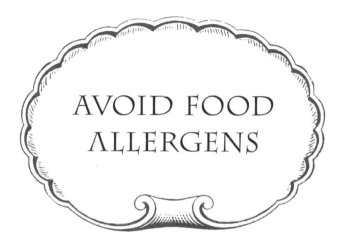

AVOID FOOD
ALLERGENS

. . . .

I like to look at all the new cookbooks and diet books
that come out. After a 30-second glance, I can tell that
many of the recipes within them contain food allergens,
and that the people who try them might develop a reaction due to food intolerance.

Removing irritating foods is one of the fastest ways
to feel energy come back into our bodies, yet most of
us don't even realize the role such allergies play in our
quest for optimal health. As we age, it's common to
develop sensitivities to environmental factors such as
grasses, pollens, dust, feathers, mold, or ragweed; but
we can also become reactive to common foods without
knowing it.

Over time, due to multiple stressors, our immune system can become compromised or overreact. Couple this

with a weak digestive tract and lack of digestive enzymes, and we have a good recipe for food intolerance—symptoms of which include fatigue, joint stiffness, digestive and respiratory problems, headaches, weight gain, and cravings. By the time we've reached the age of 60, our habits are pretty well entrenched, so the idea of giving up our favorite meals and snacks may not be appealing, but I guarantee that it's well worth it.

This chapter will illuminate all that can be gained by eliminating the items that are causing you more harm than good.

Common Food Allergies

Any good healthy-aging program should include food-allergy assessment, which is standard procedure whenever I give a reading. Unfortunately, food intolerance is very common but is nearly always misdiagnosed by traditional physicians. Food sensitivities usually stem from the items you eat on a daily basis. Think of what you consume every day—probably dairy products such as milk, yogurt, cheese, ice cream, or cottage cheese, right? Well, dairy is one of the major food allergies out there, along with wheat, corn, soy, and yeast.

Let's look at the "major offenders" in detail:

1. **Cow's milk** is the most common allergen, and many people may react poorly to products that are made from it. Symptoms include gas, bloating, bowel problems, stomach cramps, weight gain, puffy eyes, and sinus and respiratory infections.

You can substitute dairy products from cows with those from goats and sheep, for these are completely different food families and have different chemical or phenolic compositions.

2. If cow's milk is the most common allergen, then **wheat** comes in a close second. Wheat in any form can cause joint stiffness, arthritis, tiredness or exhaustion, puffiness or fluid retention, poor absorption, bowel problems, heaviness, soreness, and "heat" in the feet or ankles. The vast number of people who are afflicted with arthritis or joint stiffness could find relief by simply avoiding wheat. It doesn't matter if it's a sprouted, whole-grain, organic, or nonorganic product; wheat is an inflammatory food for many individuals, no matter what form it takes.

You can substitute wheat products with bread or crackers made of 100 percent rye, rice, quinoa, or millet —many of these "alternative" breads and crackers can be found in health-food stores.

3. For an aging person, **corn** presents two problems: (1) It is very close to sugar, and blood-sugar issues can become increasingly prevalent as the years tick by; and (2) corn can be deleterious to the digestive tract. You see, the lining of your small intestine should consist of a thick carpet of *villi*, which resemble blades of grass and are involved in the absorption of nutrition. As we age, our digestive mechanisms wear down, leading to poor absorption of nutrition—which means that nutrients from our food aren't nourishing or rebuilding our bodies.

Almost everything packaged contains corn because it's a cheap, sweet filler—it's used widely in the baking industry. If you'd like an alternative to cornstarch when you're cooking, try tapioca starch, which is available in Asian grocery stores.

4. Intuitively, I see **soy** being a problem for many people—it feels like a heavy weight when I view it in the body. Lots of individuals are legume sensitive, and since soy is a bean, it can be difficult to digest. However, men and women from Asia, India, or other cultures where generations have used soy successfully are more able to digest and assimilate it.

Soy can block the absorption of iron and B vitamins, and there's some evidence to suggest that frequent consumption may elevate estrogen levels, which can then contribute to excess weight, estrogen dominance, or breast cancer.

5. **Yeasts** are common allergens found in bread, baked products, wine, beer, and fermented foods such as vinegar, pickles, and condiments. Exposure to yeasts in a person's food, air, or environment can cause him or her to feel anxious or depressed and trigger something as simple as a runny nose!

6. As the aging stomach and digestive tract become a little more finicky, one might become sensitive to **acidic foods** such as tomatoes, citrus fruits, and spicy items. In the case of arthritis, sensitivities to the nightshade family can develop. Potatoes, tomatoes, all peppers, eggplant, and tobacco are all triggers.

7. **Sugar** and **coffee** aren't really considered to be allergens, but they do impact the nervous system. As time progresses, we want to keep our nervous system intact, as it affects our balance and clear thinking. By minimizing our intake of stimulants such as sugar, caffeine, chocolate, and alcohol, we can feel steadier, calmer, and

more relaxed. We're less likely to be distracted, forgetful, jittery, off balance, or unstable on our feet.

Arresting the Death Process

Anne called me for a consultation after her children told her that they wanted to put her into a nursing home. She was 72 years old and had been having some memory problems, yet she was adamant that she wanted to stay in the ranch house that her husband had built— the place where she'd raised her children, mowed her lawn, and planted her vegetable garden. Unfortunately, thanks to arthritis, she was no longer able to shop for groceries or tend to the garden.

I tuned in to Anne and could see that she was feisty and strong at her core, and there was lots of life left in her. I asked if she'd like to do a little experiment in food-allergy avoidance, and she said yes. After we reduced the amount of wheat and sugar in her diet, the results were pretty miraculous. Anne reported that she had more energy, could think more clearly, and her arthritis had backed off . . . best of all, she'd be able to stay in her own home.

This reminds me of a presentation I gave a few years ago at a luxurious retirement/independent living complex in Tucson, Arizona. Why I offered to do this, I don't know. I've never been so apprehensive about a speech in my whole life. *What on earth am I going to discuss with these seniors?* I thought.

When I walked up to the podium, the words seemed to come from nowhere. I talked about diet and its relationship to strength and mental clarity. I mentioned how much admiration I had for our elders and how we could all look to them for wisdom and insight. I was also sure that they'd mastered the art of forgiveness, which was something we youngsters were still working on.

I continued for the allotted 45 minutes, and completed my talk to a standing ovation. What I'd shared made sense to them even if it had been a mystery to me!

At the end of the presentation, a meticulously dressed older lady approached me and said with great intensity that she related to everything I'd said. Apparently, she'd tried an experiment a few weeks back of not eating desserts and noticed that she had more energy and could think more clearly. She'd mastered forgiveness, but once she started to resist her addictions, she got more of her life back. This woman was arresting the death process.

I want to diverge a little bit and talk about an interesting phenomenon that began years ago: I started to notice the death process on an energetic level, and I still remember my first experience in doing so. The year was 1990, and I'd come up with a special children's project called "Angels 4 Kids," which consisted of a cuddly, angel-shaped pillow and a set of healing music-and-story CDs to comfort children and assist them in getting to sleep. To date, this project has helped thousands of children around the world. (For more information on Angels 4 Kids, please see the product list in the back of this book.)

I'd finished all the scripts for the CDs, but now I needed to find someone to create the angel-shaped pillows. Through several chance encounters, I arranged to meet with a woman in Seattle who was skilled in making stuffed toys . . . and as soon as I met her, I had a foreboding sense that I've come to recognize as the death process. As it turned out, several months later this woman's husband died of a brain tumor. At the time of our meeting, neither of them had any knowledge of his impending diagnosis.

The death process is where the body is more engaged in breaking down than it is in living, and it can be a conscious or unconscious process. It's visible to me in people I meet, including an acquaintance of mine whom I recently bumped into. I hadn't seen this man in several years, and although he was only in his early 70s, I could instantly tell that he was slipping away—his precious life force was slowly moving in the direction of death.

On a higher, spiritual level, the death process is quite fascinating and can be observed intuitively. The level of energy within the body, and the desire to be fully here on the planet, will be very low. On a subconscious level, many people don't want to keep going because their existence is difficult, painful, and disappointing. They give up on life, and the death process begins.

After 25 years of working in the field of medical intuition, I believe that arresting this decay, breakdown, and death process is very important because it all relates to the notion of destiny. I consider it my spiritual task to help each person build up his or her immune system and engage the will to live so that he or she can complete that destiny. We all need to have the physical stamina and energy to finish our soul's script, because if we don't, we'll cycle out, leave the planet, and (if you believe in reincarnation) have to wait for possibly another thousand years until circumstances are right to be reborn.

It's time to wake up and get our bodies in harmony, health, and balance so that we can complete our destiny and live the life we were intended to. Our mission is to be all that we can be and to reach our full potential by staving off the body's breakdown.

The Role of Yeasts and Fungi

The breakdown and decay process is largely due to yeast, bacteria, parasites, and fungi living off the body. What most interests me is a strain of yeast called *Candida albicans,* which naturally occurs in human beings. It can be located in the digestive tract, lungs, sinuses, skin, mouth, nose, urethra, genitals, blood, or brain; and everyone from a baby to a grandparent can be dealing with an overgrowth of this ubiquitous strain of yeast. In fact, if you ever visit (let's hope it's only a visit) a nursing home, you'll be met at the door by a distinct smell— this is the scent of yeast, or the death process. All of the people at that nursing home have made a subconscious decision to gather there and wait to die.

As soon as I detect yeast, which has a sickly sweet odor, I know that a body is breaking down. The person may be experiencing fatigue or memory loss, suffering from lung or breathing problems, dealing with skin patches or psoriasis, or experiencing uncontrollable cravings.

In a healthy person, Candida albicans, other strains of yeast, and fungi exist in balance with normal intestinal flora or bacteria. Healthy flora is necessary for digestion, assimilation of nutrition, and the prevention of infection. Yet under certain conditions, especially in the case of a weakened immune system, Candida yeast can increase rapidly and overtake the normal, beneficial gut bacteria. This is largely due to the Western world's overuse of antibiotics, the side effects of birth control pills, and our dependence on starch- and sugar-laden diets. The gut flora becomes imbalanced, and the yeast is allowed to proliferate out of control.

I was diagnosed with Candida yeast in an overgrowth state myself when I was 39 years old. Arresting this syndrome, which was systemic (that is, throughout my system) at the time, gave me back my energy, vitality, and mental clarity. This is what I want for you, too.

Many people think that yeast is a woman's issue, but men are just as susceptible to Candida. To me, this is the "missing piece" that everyone must be mindful of in his or her ongoing health program. The core of a healthy-aging plan is going to involve eradicating this yeast . . . and the death process.

The death process is similar to what happens to a tree in the forest. Perhaps you've taken a walk and noticed a large white fungus growing off the side of a tree trunk—this fungal growth is robbing that tree of its vital energy. The tree becomes weak and infested with vermin, and it eventually falls over and dies. This is part of the life cycle . . . but *you* don't need to fall before your time.

When yeasts, fungi, parasites, or bacteria are present in the body, its immune system and natural defenses become compromised. Then the body eventually breaks down and is overtaken by the organisms within it. Candida albicans in a prolific state is the beginning of death to the human being, so don't be such a nice host to the yeast or fungus that lives inside you.

Still Trendy after All These Years

The yeast syndrome was very trendy in the 1980s, and the most well-known book written about the subject was *The Yeast Connection: A Medical Breakthrough* (Vintage), by William Crook, a medical doctor from Tennessee. "Billy Crook," as he was fondly called, brought the subject to light—and of course he was pooh-poohed by the medical establishment, even though thousands of professional articles had been written about candidiasis. When Crook died just a few years ago, he'd barely scratched the surface of educating the public about this important subject.

How would you know if you were dealing with Candida yeast in an overgrowth state? Well, you'd probably be tired and crave sweets. You might also be experiencing memory loss and wondering if you had the beginnings of Alzheimer's. These are all telltale signs.

It's interesting to note that almost all major diseases—from cancer to AIDS, multiple sclerosis, chronic fatigue syndrome, and Alzheimer's disease—have Candida albicans as part of their symptom profiles. Many nurses also report to me that Candida is listed on patients' charts, yet nothing is done in the hospital to treat it.

One look at advertising will let you know that the prevalence of Candida albicans has grown to epidemic proportions, at least in North America: Note all the television commercials for products targeting toenail fungus, psoriasis, eczema, dandruff, rectal itching, vaginal yeast infections, bladder frequency, or even memory function. This is not a mystery—it's all about arresting the death process, and the yeast syndrome is an important link to these irritating problems. In the case of psoriasis, topical skin preparations are only a temporary solution, as Candida needs to be eradicated internally. That's where the major health and anti-aging work begins: on the inside of your body.

The Sugar/Aging Connection

I find it interesting that every element in health is interrelated. For example, sugary things, including starch and alcohol, feed the yeast that contributes to body breakdown and disease. While I'd long suspected that there was a connection between sugar and aging, it took Ron Rosedale, M.D.—author (along with Carol Colman) of *The Rosedale Diet: Turn off Your Hunger Switch* (HarperCollins)—to confirm it for me.

According to Rosedale, longevity and animal studies show that the crucial marker for a longer life span is insulin sensitivity or low insulin levels. So if your insulin levels are high, your blood-glucose levels will be higher than they should be. When glucose (sugar) levels are elevated, your body switches from cell regeneration and repair into cell reproduction and proliferation—this is the important link to cancer growth.

Foods that raise sugar and insulin levels will be stored as fat, thus putting pressure on the heart. Insulin is also a growth hormone, so when our bodies are bombarded by it, we can develop prediabetes, hyperinsulinemia, or insulin resistance. This means that cells stop responding to insulin, and cell damage, cell breakdown, and cancer-cell proliferation can occur. The first effect of insulin resistance is excess weight gain, followed by obesity, then diabetes, and possibly cancer. According to Dr.

Rosedale, sugary foods—even fruit—can promote cancer growth.

Glycation (glucose reacting with protein) causes inflammation, memory problems, nerve-cell injury, age spots, wrinkles, and premature aging. Although this process occurs in everyone, it does so at higher rates for those with elevated blood sugar—that is, diabetics and prediabetics. Dr. Rosedale explains that these are the people who suffer the diseases of aging, since the longest-living animals and humans have consistently low blood-sugar levels for their age.

A simple way to stop glycation is to lay off sugars and refined carbohydrates, and instead ingest the complex carbohydrates found in vegetables and whole grains. This practical concept of reducing sugars and starch was brought home to me in 1998, when I embraced the concept of lowering my intake of carbs. At that time I was in my mid-50s and had started to put on weight as the result of declining hormones. I was looking for a solution, and it didn't take long for it to come to me.

Friends introduced me to the work of Michael and Mary Dan Eades, two medical doctors from Boulder, Colorado, whose groundbreaking book, *Protein Power: The High-Protein/Low-Carbohydrate Way to Lose Weight, Feel Fit, and Boost Your Health—in Just Weeks!* (Bantam), dramatically changed the direction of my health.

The Eades' work is based on the concept that decreasing starches and sugars can reduce weight and lower blood pressure and cholesterol. They've been very successful in helping people recover from these health issues strictly by changing their diets. I, too, lost my excess weight and regained more energy as soon as I lowered my intake of carbs. (Visit: **www.proteinpower.com**.)

An understanding of carbohydrate metabolism will assist you in implementing this kind of plan.

Carbohydrate Metabolism

Everything you eat consists of water; fats; protein; and carbohydrates, which are forms of starch and sugar. A few years ago the low-carbohydrate diet was very popular, thanks to the *New Diet Revolution,* a book by cardiologist and nutritionist Robert C. Atkins, M.D. Atkins was soundly criticized for his findings that a diet low in sugar and starch could lower cholesterol and blood pressure and balance the blood sugars of diabetic and prediabetic patients. Yet the whole notion of eating heartily while still dieting was a welcome relief to so many people, and the craze caught on. Finally, the American Heart Association recognized that a plan like Dr. Atkins's could indeed be beneficial.

A few years after Dr. Atkins died from accidental causes, the low-carb fad fizzled out. Maybe it was because Dr. Atkins had really left his mark, so the banner could then continue to be carried by the people who understood and appreciated its principles. But I think that there are some inherent issues in the low-carbohydrate diet that make it difficult for most individuals to follow in the long term—the traditional program focuses on high protein, very few fruits or vegetables, lots of dairy products (which are a common allergen), and many processed and chemically laden packaged snack foods.

Although some people can be very successful on a low-carbohydrate diet, in the long run it can lead to an overloaded liver and gallbladder, as well as some very poor eating habits. In addition, packaged foods are expensive and may contain ingredients and chemicals to which your body could negatively react, thus sabotaging successful weight loss. Such foods often contain soy protein, for instance, which can affect the thyroid function that's necessary for fat-burning metabolism, or whey, a dairy derivative and common irritant.

The body functions better on a well-balanced diet. So go ahead and choose the elements of a low-carb program, but eat healthy foods, too. The basic principle behind a low-carbohydrate plan is that you avoid or greatly reduce starches such as breads, pasta, cakes, cookies, corn, rice, potatoes, or sugar. The idea is to keep carbohydrate grams from these starches and sugars low— approximately 30 to 60 grams a day. Then, as weight loss takes place and insulin levels normalize, additional grams can be added. There is no limit to the amount of green, leafy vegetables you can consume on a daily basis.

Carbohydrates and Cholesterol

People always ask me why carbohydrates are involved in cholesterol production but proteins and fats aren't. Well, the pancreas releases insulin to take care of the rise in blood sugar that's caused by carbs; and at the same time, it gives a message to the liver to create cholesterol to match the amount of insulin released.

It goes like this: "Hi, liver, this is me, pancreas. Say, Bob/Mary just put down a bowl of cereal, a glass of juice, and a banana for breakfast. We've got a big rise in insulin here because of that high-carb breakfast, so can you make cholesterol to match that insulin?"

70

The liver replies, "Okay, pancreas, I'll get right on it."

So the plan is to keep the starches and sugars low so that your pancreas isn't constantly giving the liver the signal to create cholesterol. By stopping these insulin spikes, your cholesterol will return to normal levels very quickly.

Let's turn to my 81-year-old friend Bonnie, whom I discussed earlier. For years she had problems trying to get her cholesterol levels down to normal. She'd been avoiding offending foods but made the mistake of eating too much millet, brown rice, and alternative grains with her meals. I introduced her to the low-carb diet, subtracting the grains but adding a lot more vegetables. She was delighted to see the dramatic drop in cholesterol levels after only one month, something that had eluded her for many years. Even her doctor was impressed.

The Metaphysics of Blood-Sugar Metabolism

My mother was a dietitian, and she made sure we had a hearty breakfast every morning—one that always included eggs. I'm greatly concerned about the number of people who start their days with coffee (also hard on the pancreas), a glass of juice, and a piece of toast, without one speck of protein. No wonder diabetes is becoming an epidemic.

Here's a fascinating look at the metaphysical or causal side of poor sugar handling. I find it interesting that type 2 diabetes is an "adult" onset disease, when no adult has actually been present! Your adult side, who should be looking out for you, taking care of you, and attending to your physical body's needs, has in effect been absent. Your childish side, which has given in to addictions and sugary temptations, has been leading the show.

This type of diabetes, with its out-of-control desires for sweets and sweetness from life, can reflect a strong-willed inner child. So why not reorient that inner child toward some creativity? Focus on your goals and dreams, and discover what mark you'd like to leave on the planet. As soon as you feel happy and fulfilled in your soul's purpose, you'll have no need to placate yourself with food or drink. You *will* get there—you'll realize that discipline regarding what you consume and your health is an important step in climbing your mountain of personal self-mastery.

Since we've thoroughly explored the "big three" reasons for the breakdown of our physical house, let's move our focus to emotions.

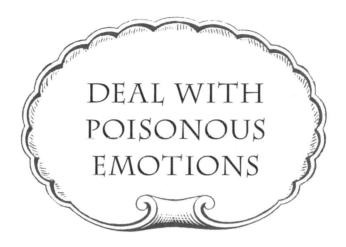

CHAPTER 6

DEAL WITH POISONOUS EMOTIONS

Toxicity can come in an emotional package as well as a physical one. A perfect example of this is a woman named Janice, whom I met at a glamorous spa. I was there for a few days giving presentations, and as I sat next to her at dinner, I intuitively noticed that she was on a number of medications.

It turns out that Janice was at the spa for a few days of reflection, a gift to herself for her 57th birthday. She'd been married for 20 years to a man who verbally abused her—he continually belittled her and often loudly criticized or judged her in front of their 18-year-old son. He also had complete control over her emotions and the family finances. It had gotten to the point where she felt so beaten down that her immune system had begun to overreact. She was now on several medications, including three antidepressants and pills for anxiety.

Janice felt that she was at a critical turning point in her life and was examining her choices and options, both to recover her physical strength and her mental well-being. As we talked over dinner, she told me that she thought a miracle had arrived at her table—and in a way, perhaps it had.

I immediately grabbed a piece of paper and started writing down some simple guidelines to strengthen her immune system and detoxify her body. One aspect of the game plan was to work on Janice's liver: I explained that all the medications she was taking would have toxic effects on that organ, so I suggested some detoxification herbs, a lot of raw vegetables, and plenty of water. The real toxic examination, however, related to her relationship, which was taking her very essence away from her.

Power Leakage

Why do people stay in a fire? The clothes they're wearing are burning, but they stay in the flames, hoping that things will cool down and life will be peaceful. After 20 years with one cruel person, this was obviously not going to happen . . . it was time to move on.

Here was a beautiful, personable, and intelligent professional woman who could make her way in the world perfectly well, yet Janice was staying in a toxic relationship that was breaking her heart and her spirit. Valuable energy was draining out of her body because of it, and it was destroying her soul as well. Her will to live was damaged, and save for a level of core strength that she seemed to possess, she was teetering on the brink of giving up on life. At a time like this, with her body's resources stretched thin, cancer could be an unwelcome guest.

Would this woman be ready to climb the mountain and claim her own life, or would she be content to circle the perimeter? I wholeheartedly prayed for the former.

Just like Janice, many men and women are mired in toxic relationships, which can age them as quickly as poisonous drugs and substances can. Such patterns go way back: For women, they could stem from a controlling, dominant father; while for men, they might point to a mother issue. As children, we were programmed to stay quiet—we weren't supposed to rock the boat or make Mommy or Daddy mad, so we learned to suppress our emotions. Because we hold on to patterns, as we get older we invariably magnetize to ourselves a person who exactly mirrors what we believe on the inside.

For a graphic look at where energy and power is leaking out of your body, take out a pen and a piece of paper and follow these steps:

1. Imagine that you're a large oblong container of energy.

2. See that there are cords running out of your container.

3. Visualize each one of these cords plugged into your job, your relationship, your children, your elderly parent, your finances, and so forth.

4. Take a look at this picture closely. Now draw what your container looks like, along with the cords and each issue they're plugged into.

5. Place your hand on your heart and ask yourself how much of your energy is invested in your relationship. Write down the answer.

6. Repeat the question for each of the "drains" you've jotted down. Keep in mind that if 60 percent of your energy is going to your children, then you only have 40 percent going to your job, your mate, and you!

I like to think of energy as little suitcases with feet, which run away from the body. A daily examination of your energy loss will help you to better control it: For example, you'll see that chocolate and coffee negatively impact your body on the physical level; constantly dwelling on a past issue saps your body's strength emotionally; and staying with someone who doesn't value or support you will damage you spiritually.

It's time to change the belief system. You've been told that you're "a beloved child of God" . . . what does that mean? Well, you are a son or daughter of the universe and have a right to be here, and you need to claim that right. As you come to believe in this deep truth and make all of your decisions based upon it, you'll be less likely to allow anyone who is toxic or damaging into your life.

Lack and Limitation

The story of a woman named Elaine illustrates the connection between energy and draining situations, plus the important element of lack. She told me that the energy flooded back into her body once she made the decision to leave her husband some years ago. She'd entered the marriage as a wealthy woman with great confidence and independence, along with a high spirit. Decades of rearing children, running a household, and dealing with her husband's risky business ventures (for which he used *her* money) had worn her down, and she decided it was time to cut loose.

Now in her mid-90s, Elaine is in impressive physical shape. Distance swimming in the master's category is her passion, and she can beat most of the 80-year-olds. What's her secret? Good genes, daily exercise, and financial security—after all, nothing will take down energy and vitality faster than the feeling of lack.

Take Nick and Pam, for example. This couple thought they'd adequately prepared for retirement, but Nick lost his job at age 59 when his company went bankrupt, and he lost his pension as well. Since Nick and Pam hadn't anticipated this, their lives were thrown into a virtual tailspin. They seemed to age overnight: Nick's hair went pure white, and Pam changed from being radiant to looking lined and drawn. When they examined their "energy-storage containers," they found that 90 percent of their energy was draining out in worry over finances.

Don't let this happen to you. Wherever you are now in life, plan ahead! Your feelings of independence, confidence, and self-esteem depend on being in charge—of your feelings, your body, and your finances. Don't make the mistake of thinking that your spouse or company will take care of you and that your pension is secure. These are very different times.

This brings to mind Vern, who called in to one of my teleconferences to ask about rectal bleeding. (**Note:**

Rectal bleeding is a serious thing, so if it's happening to you, see your medical doctor for a consultation and probably a colonoscopy immediately! Colon problems or colorectal cancer can be detected and treated, so be proactive.)

As I spoke to Vern, I had a sense that he had suffered a financial setback. This was indeed the case: He'd worked in the automobile industry for 35 years, and at age 67, he'd been living off his pension for two years. He thought that his pension plan was secure, but thanks to a company reshuffle, it had been reduced by a third. All of a sudden, he was thrust into the unknown—and a state of panic.

Over the years, Vern had suffered from constipation, and now because of the stress, he was experiencing bouts of rectal bleeding. These were my strategies for him:

— On the emotional level, the colon represents the elimination process, including letting go of the past and old ideas or outmoded beliefs, and the blood represents the "chi" or life force, or the amount of energy one has invested in oneself or others. Vern's belief that his pension was the only source of income was the issue at hand. On a practical level, this could be the truth; but on a higher level, there were other options yet to be seen . . . scary, but exciting, too!

This current experience was an important opportunity for Vern's growth and a "way in" to developing trust. I let him know that the well-known adage "What is in the way—is the way" could help him understand that his bleeding rectum, energy leakage toward the past, and fear of the future were providing him with a catalyst to move in a new direction.

One way to get the healing energy back into Vern's body was to work on forgiveness: toward his company *and* himself, for the choices they both made. After all, on a higher level, he "set it up this way" for his growth and learning. No, forgiveness isn't an easy task, but the rewards are numerous, including more energy in the body, deeper and lighter meditations, and the space for change to take place.

— On the physical level, I gave Vern some hints to keep his bowels moving and the energy flowing, such as to increase his intake of green, leafy vegetables. A good-sized salad at lunch and dinner can work wonders. (I like to make one for myself that's "fully loaded" with all sorts of greens, seeds, shredded cabbage, and fibrous vegetables.) Adding olive, flax, or other vegetable oils can be useful because it coats the intestinal tract so that stools "slip" through the GI tract more easily. I had Vern try two tablespoons a day, either "straight up" or poured onto his salads.

I also had him increase the amount of whole grains in his diet—including some unusual ones like quinoa, millet, and amaranth. I told him to be sure that his water intake was high, at least eight glasses per day.

— Finally, I asked Vern to develop his faith by repeating the comforting affirmation *I have faith in my future.* Because he needed to think about building a life centered on his own gifts and talents, I mentioned that a good counselor or strategist could help identify his skills and point him in a new direction. Everyone has something to offer, so Vern needed to be open to all opportunities. I reminded him that the universe really wants to deliver good to us . . . we just need to believe it.

Long-Term Care Insurance

Preventing the dispersion of your own personal power is an ongoing feat of self-mastery. Often, you'll be dealing with issues that are beyond your control—for example, as much as you love and want to help your elderly parent, this could be draining your power and energy reserves. If he or she has Alzheimer's disease, for instance, it presents a big financial concern. And on top of that, there are extra chores, shopping, and doctors' appointments for you to take care of, which can be exhausting and worrying.

Thanks to modern medicine, our parents are living longer . . . which isn't always a good thing if their quality of life is significantly diminished. It frightens us to see them deteriorate and to be faced with the question of how long we might be dealing with the complications. While I'm sure that each one of us has made a silent vow not to end up in this state, now is the time to prepare for the future so that we're taken care of and don't become burdens ourselves.

If we look after ourselves and make the necessary lifestyle choices, with a piece of luck we may not need long-term care (LTC) insurance. But as the saying goes, "Believe in Allah, but tie your camel," so investigating this option makes sense.

LTC insurance policies differ widely: Some of them pay for up to three years of care with no consideration for what might happen down the line; some don't kick in until the person has been in a facility for up to three months, and companies may be suspect in not honoring claims because the insured parties are too old to navigate their way through some of the policy's obstacles. Long-term care is a gamble between you and the insurance company. Will you even need it, and will the company actually pay if you do? I hear that complaints about this type of insurance rose more than 90 percent from 2001 to 2006, mostly because of claim denials.

Apparently, the odds are in the insurers' favor, since many people in their 50s and 60s who purchase the insurance never make a claim—but that's a good thing. Do read the fine print, as the initial premiums can be low, only to escalate as a person ages. That's exactly what happened to Ellen and Max, who purchased LTC insurance when they were both 56. They thought it was a good idea at the time, but it's now ten years later, their premiums have increased 40 percent, and they feel locked into something they can no longer afford. They can continue to pay the premiums and not end up using the insurance, or they can cancel the policy now and throw thousands of dollars in premiums down the drain.

It's time for you to do some planning. Do you own your home? Do you have resources if you require long-term care? (Of course, if you live in Canada, medical insurance and long-term housing and care are all available to any permanent resident regardless of means.)

Special Issues for Women

Practical realities can hit hard. Did you know that 60 million women in the United States are living without spouses? Yet that doesn't have to be the end for them. Here's a story on this subject that I find very inspirational.

When Lorna's husband, Dale, died, she went to work because she knew that she couldn't live on the pension or life-insurance policy he'd left her—at age 62, she took matters into her own hands. Although she'd been a wife, mother, and homemaker for her entire life, she had a talent for baking. As she was also an early riser, she applied at the local bakery to work part-time. Soon Lorna was turning out breads, muffins, and scones; and after a few months, she authored a cookbook. While the recipes in it aren't that healthy, in my estimation, Lorna has created her own recipe for health and happiness. She was willing to dive in and support herself rather than worry each month about paying her bills, and she loves her job and the new life she's made for herself.

It's predicted that seven out of ten women who are now age 60 will outlive their husbands, and 30 percent of 65-year-old women are expected to live to age 90. So if we're 60 now, we have some planning to do, particularly since women traditionally fall short in financial planning for their retirement. I have visions of my widowed grandmother in her little apartment in Edinburgh, Scotland, existing on toast and tea until she was put into a "home."

According to statistics, older women have less money in their savings accounts than their male counterparts do, and the typical balance in a female's retirement savings plan or 401(k) is 40 percent lower than a male's. That's why so many women reinvent themselves several times before the age of 60, especially if they've been stay-at-home wives and mothers for most of their lives.

My mother faced this fact when she was widowed at age 57, with a 13-year-old son to raise. She reviewed the pension options that were left to her by my father and decided that she needed to go back to work. She had a teacher's credential and recent experience teaching English as a second language, so she took a refresher course and went to work at a local community college. Although she mourned the recent death of her soul mate, teaching new immigrants gave her a purpose, and she was able to raise her son with fewer financial worries.

I recommend the following books for my fellow women, since these authors will propel you into thinking practically and creatively about your financial future:

- *The Feminine Mistake: Are We Giving Up Too Much?* by Leslie Bennetts

- *Nice Girls Don't Get Rich: 75 Avoidable Mistakes Women Make with Money,* by Lois P. Frankel, Ph.D.

- *Women & Money: Owning the Power to Control Your Destiny,* by Suze Orman

Now let's assess the management of your own personal power. Answer yes or no to the following questions:

- Do you worry about your future?

- Do you believe that others are more adept, intelligent, or capable than you are?

- Do you dwell on past issues and wish that you could have made different choices?

- Do you have stomach or digestive issues?

- Do you have friends or family members who are negative or hurtful to you?

I spent 21 years as a wife, mother, and homemaker, until my world fell apart. I then took my meager divorce settlement and started again. After asking myself the preceding questions and really paying attention to the answers, I decided to invest in myself. Anyone else would have played it safe, but I did not. I didn't have a plan, but I did have my inner compass, which led me to explore my full potential. I've taken big risks, but it's all worked out. Thanks to 25 years of listening to my inner guidance and using my intuition, I've carved out a very fulfilling life for myself. I'm now living my soul's purpose—something that others only dream about.

If *you* are willing to use your gifts and talents to carve out your own niche, no one can take that away from you. You'll have created your own brand; and no boss, merger, or pension default could ever rob you of that. I urge more women—and men—to explore their creative potential.

Naturally, paddling your own canoe can be pretty stressful at times, especially when you're creating "a job out of the ethers." It seems ironic that I have a number of best-selling relaxation CD programs—the expression "you teach what you need to learn" very often applies to me.

I have a lot of stress in my life as an author and speaker, because there are numerous deadlines for books, articles, and speeches. While my life is fun, varied, and purposeful, finding the balance with my "driven" nature can be elusive at times. Consequently, these are my favorite ways to de-stress:

- Boating out on the ocean

- Swimming

- Meditating, usually next to the water

- Soaking in a hot bath before bed

- Sleeping, including taking a power nap when necessary

- Rocking in a chair with a good book

- Taking short, relaxing breaks

- Holding my precious grandchildren

- Eating a good diet that keeps blood sugars balanced

- Supplementing with specific nutrients, B vitamins, and adrenal support

I urge you to find your own ways to decompress and use them often.

Forming a Healing Alliance

Lowering stress helps us live longer, and forming a healing alliance will help with that process. But first I'd like to take a minute to talk about supplements.

Many people have a poor diet and take too many vitamins—every time a symptom appears, they trundle off to the nearest store for a bottle of pills. The body digests and processes food efficiently; therefore, you'll get the best result when you look for food-based supplements to augment your nutrition. The body doesn't have the capacity to digest or utilize synthesized or manufactured supplements, so many supplements that are foreign to the body just end up becoming expensive urine.

A family-owned company called Standard Process, of Palmyra, Wisconsin, has been in the business of producing glandular and food-based supplements since 1930. Standard Process's founder, Royal Lee, was a dentist with a great interest in nutrition who discovered that if he gave people ground-up vegetables (or even pulverized animal parts) pressed into capsules, they got well.

Personally, I experienced a big jump in my energy and vitality when I began using this company's products in 1998, and I'm very grateful to my Seattle practitioners for introducing them to me. Most chiropractors in the United States use Standard Process supplements, but please note that they're professional formulas that aren't sold in health-food stores. (Please visit: **www. standardprocess.com.**)

The following make up a good anti-aging supplement regimen—note that they should all be food based when appropriate:

- An all-vegetable multiple vitamin

- Absorbable calcium

- Digestive enzymes

- 500 mg of Ester-C

- Fish oils such as cod-liver or krill oil

- Vegetable oils such as flax and borage

- Probiotics

- Supplements to eradicate Candida yeast

- Bioidentical hormones, if needed

- Specific supplements recommended by your naturopath, holistic medical doctor, or nutritionist

Keep pills to a minimum, and get most of your nutritional value from organic, healthy foods. Your own intuition can play an important role in determining which supplement, herb, or botanical will be beneficial for you and promote a vibrant-aging program. I also strongly recommend that you follow up with a good local practitioner. You and this person, along with your medical doctor, will become the primary members of your healing team.

The best practitioners are the ones you hear about through word of mouth—after all, success needs to be shared. Consult with someone who looks healthy and exudes vibrant pure energy, one who "walks the walk and talks the talk." Choose a good naturopathic physician or a holistic M.D. who does foundation nutritional work as well as comprehensive blood or saliva testing.

After you've changed your diet and picked out your supplements, your next step is foundation support for your liver, kidneys, adrenals, heart, and digestive system.

This is where an acupuncturist can be helpful. Acupuncture is nothing to be frightened of, since the application of the needles is virtually painless. The practice can do wonders for pain management, headaches, stopping addictions, boosting energy, and alleviating countless other complaints. Again, acupuncture treatments or your alternative practitioner's methods will be infinitely more effective if you're following a healthy diet—that's the baseline.

When looking at the whole body, your alternative-practitioner list should include a massage therapist or bodyworker. He or she will help release blocked energy and symptoms on the emotional as well as physical levels.

Another form of healing that can be very useful is energy work. Many naturopathic physicians are utilizing this "biofeedback therapy," which uses subtle energies to test and heal.

In the next chapter, you'll learn how to do your own testing.

CHAPTER 7

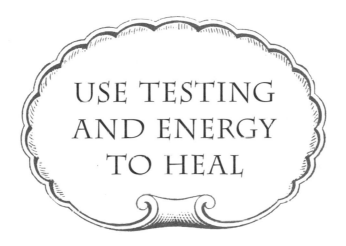

USE TESTING
AND ENERGY
TO HEAL

. . . .

I know that all of the information you've been taking in here can be pretty overwhelming. It's natural to
be asking, "But how does this apply to me?"

You're an individual, so what's best for you isn't
necessarily right for someone else. Therefore, it doesn't
really matter what anyone else tells you or what any
book says—what matters is what your *body* is trying to
tell you. You can improve your looks on the outside, but
your focus must be on the inside, which is where aging
is really taking place.

In my book *The Body "Knows,"* I describe several
methods of self-testing that enable you to maximize
your body's messages. For example, if your hands feel
stiff after you drink iced tea, you'll want to know if it's
the caffeine in the tea, the chemicals in the tea mixture,

or the sugar in the beverage that's causing the reaction. The techniques in this chapter will help you find the answers to these questions and more.

I'm a firm believer in teaching you the way to help yourself. Get your power back and become your own healer . . . after all, the body knows.

Tuning in with a Pendulum

There's no better way to discover your own health truth than by using a pendulum, or a weighted object that can give you a yes or no answer to questions. Pendulums have been used for hundreds of years as common "dowsing" tools.

Every year, dowsing conferences take place around the world, and groups of fascinating men and women gather to discuss their latest findings. (For more information on dowsing, visit: **www.dowsingtips.com**.) Dowsers are very skilled, tuned-in people whom large mining and oil companies hire to locate oil or mineral stores on maps—using pendulums or forked sticks, they wait for their tools to quiver or bend over the elements being searched for, or they might feel the quality of the terrain change as they move from one area to another. When they achieve a positive result, chances are that what they've responded to on the map will then be found in the actual geographical location.

While dowsing is a gift, anyone can learn it. I've taught thousands of people this way of tuning in, including veterinarians, who dowse for imbalances in their animal patients. I have a couple of engineer clients who use a pendulum over everything they eat. These are skilled individuals who are involved in huge building projects around the world, yet they rely upon their instincts to tell them which foods are beneficial for them. Through this method, they've learned what their bodies really want, thus removing any guesswork. It warms my heart to think of them with pendulums poised over their breakfasts each morning.

As you choose your own pendulum, be sure that it's heavy enough to drop down and hang, like a weight from a chain or string. If the weight is too light, it may not swing successfully—it may flip around and not give you a straight answer. You can find metal or crystal pendulums at health-food stores or self-help bookstores; or you can make your own out of a medallion on a chain, a piece of string or thread looped through a ring, or a common nut that you can buy at any hardware store. If you loop a short piece of soft string (approximately 16 inches long) through the nut, this makes a perfect pendulum.

I have many clients who lovingly "ask the nut" for wisdom and guidance when they want to know the benefits of a supplement or a food. As a woman I spoke to the other day in Albany, New York, told me, "When I can't find my husband, I know he'll be in the den, asking the nut."

Let's give it a try!

Welcome to Pendulum 101

Using a pendulum will help you sense or identify a response to questions regarding your own body, thus allowing you to become familiar with what it really wants. Your desire here is to know the truth *for you:*

Don't concern yourself with what others have said or what books have told you, but instead focus on what your body wants to tell you. To be able to tap into this knowing is a great gift—one that gives you power and control over your health choices.

Please keep in mind that a pendulum can only respond with a yes or no answer to your questions; therefore, you must frame them accordingly. It's also important that you take a few deep breaths to clear your mind and center yourself before you begin, as a quiet mind can receive clear, accurate answers. Finally, be sure that you're adequately rested and hydrated when you're testing—if you're tired or thirsty, your answers are less likely to be correct.

Here's how to start communicating with your body:

- In your dominant hand, hold your pendulum between your pinched thumb and forefinger so that the weight hangs directly down from your chain or string. (Note that there should be approximately six inches of string or chain length between your fingers and the weight at the end.) Make sure that your elbow is supported on a table or counter.

- Without moving the pendulum on your own, make the request: "Show me a yes." Remember, you're asking the wisdom of your body to respond, and you're looking for a clear indication or movement in any direction. Your responses will be more accurate if you don't use your rational mind, since it will try to control or influence your pendulum's responses.

- Again, say, "Show me a yes." Concentrate on the weighted object at the end of your pendulum, for your intention is to be shown what a yes response looks like by its movement. Most likely, your pendulum will respond by either moving back and forth or going around in a circle.

- Next, make the request: "Show me a no." Concentrate fully on the pendulum, and with the intention in your mind and heart, ask it to show you what a no looks like by a different movement.

- Staying centered and calm, again say, "Show me a no." You want the pendulum to respond with a different action or movement from when it showed you a yes. Perhaps it will give you a counterclockwise circle or a back-and-forth movement. (When I demonstrate the use of the pendulum, my yes is a circle, and my no is back-and-forth movement.)

- Keep focusing, and continue to practice establishing your yes or no responses so that you're familiar with them.

As soon as you feel comfortable with your yes and no responses, you're ready to ask practical questions. First, start with what you eat most often, such as eggs, flour, orange juice, milk, cheese, sugar, salt, coffee, corn (popcorn), beans, bananas, lettuce, butter, jam, chicken, beef, or bacon. Also, bring out any fruit, vegetable, or condiment. Place them all on the kitchen or dining-room table.

The next step is to prop your elbow on the table and hold your pendulum over each item, one at a time, and ask your body's wisdom the following question: "Is this substance beneficial for my body?" (Note that "Can I eat this?" is not the right question, because you *can* eat anything, even though it might not be beneficial for you to do so.)

Check the response from your pendulum: Is it swinging back and forth, or does it want to make a circle? Some people find that the pendulum may quiver or stay still in response to a no, but if yours is doing this, it could be showing you a *maybe* response. Reframe your question and try again.

Continue questioning, "Is this substance beneficial for my body?" for each of the items on the table until you *know* which ones are beneficial and which ones aren't. After you've tested each food, set the beneficial ones aside.

Keep on testing, this time with all of your supplements. You can also test your laundry detergent, cosmetics, shampoos, pillow, or air-conditioning filter. Many times such things can be loaded with unhealthful chemicals, dust, or mold.

Points to Think About

Remember that your body only knows the answer to questions posed in present time, such as those about common foods, environmental factors, or supplements. Resist the temptation to ask about the future, since none of us can be sure of what lies ahead. Don't inquire about marrying the person next door, where you'll live next year, or when you're going to take a trip, as no one knows these things for sure. The wisdom of your body will tell you what is appropriate and beneficial *in the present moment.* Leave future issues out of your questioning.

Please keep in mind that it can take about three days of frequent pendulum use in order to become skilled enough to trust it, so don't give up or become frustrated. Most people become accurate very quickly, but others find the pendulum laborious and slow, so they prefer another form of dowsing called "muscle testing" or kinesiology, which I illustrate in *The Body "Knows."*

Ultimately, your goal is to achieve intuitive accuracy about your physical body without the use of any of these tools. Your quest is to become so instinctive about your body that you know the answer to a question almost before you ask it—which will happen when you develop your own gift of medical intuition.

You're going to love tuning in to your body in this way.

Healing Frequencies

As you progress on your healing journey, you'll begin to tap into subtle energy frequencies. Through the use of a pendulum (or any other self-testing method) and its response to your questions, you'll become aware of the subtle distinctions between what feels right and what doesn't.

Everything has a resonating frequency: The tomato that you had for lunch; the steak you ate for dinner; the chair you sit upon; the flowers, the wind, the trees, and the water all around you vibrate. And this principle of resonance is behind the theory of particle or quantum physics.

All living or inanimate objects are made up of moving particles that are vibrating at various frequencies, so when you place your hands on someone with the intent of healing, the current or frequency carries energy that is felt by him or her. Positive thoughts vibrate at higher frequencies than negative ones do.

Just try being around a negative person for a while and see what happens to the cells in your body— everything starts vibrating at a lower frequency. But if you connect with a positive person who's full of excitement and zest for life, you'll soon be excited yourself, and so will your cells. Your desire is to work on your emotional, spiritual, and physical health so that your body constantly vibrates at these higher frequencies. You'll be able to develop the level of awareness to instantly discern whenever your frequency changes or slows down, as well as what you can do about it.

In my clinical days as an allergy-testing technician, the equipment I used measured frequencies. I'd put food samples to be tested in a circuit with the patient, and the resonating frequency would tell me if there was a problem with that particular substance or not. Not only would it give me an accurate read on imbalances, the equipment could tell me the precise degree of allergy or sensitivity. This was a fascinating introduction to the world of medical intuition, and I still rely upon these subtle nuances to read imbalances in the body.

In environmental medicine, we utilized hundreds of liquid neutralizing compounds to treat patients for all kinds of metabolic problems such as food allergies, hormone imbalances, environmental factors, vitamin and mineral deficiencies, or neurotransmitter imbalances. These neutralizing compounds carried very high frequencies that were palpable. In fact, sometimes I'd just walk past the carts carrying the healing remedies and feel the strong energy they emitted. I knew that they were healing substances, which is why they were so effective.

To this day, I work with a laboratory that produces these kinds of remedies—some of which are actually my own formulas, which have come to me in meditation. Exactly how the biochemist in the lab created these is quite interesting, as their resonating frequencies match the harmonics of musical notes. Since certain kinds of music set to specific keys carry a healing frequency, vibrational remedies can be created to match those particular keys.

We need to be open to the idea of frequencies, since they can put us in touch with higher octaves of feeling and understanding. For example, years ago I heard an audiotape of the sound of crickets. You know, the "chirp, chirp" that's enough to drive you crazy at night if you're camping. But when the sound of one cricket was multiplied a thousand times, stretched out, and electronically synthesized, it was deeply compelling and seemed to impart a hidden message to me. I can't tell you what the message was, but it did carry a healing frequency that touched me deeply.

There are hidden messages in many things. I believe that these can be spiritual activators that heal cells, set events in motion, warn us of impending danger, or guide us on our path. The key is to be open to these messages . . . which happens when we keep our vibrational frequency high.

We can do this when we're having fun, dancing, or being creative; such activities keep our cells vibrating at higher levels, thus protecting us from diseases of a lower vibration. The qualities of love and happiness carry a high vibration, and we can radiate this frequency to our own bodies. This helps us regenerate and repair—which is the next topic for discussion.

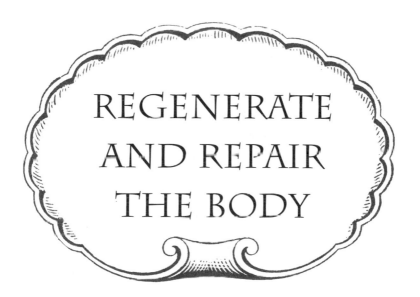

PART II

REGENERATE
AND REPAIR
THE BODY

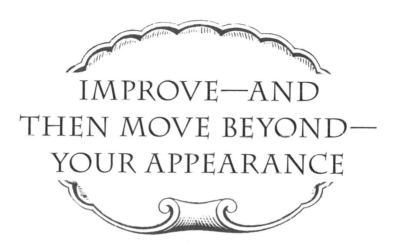

CHAPTER 8

IMPROVE—AND THEN MOVE BEYOND— YOUR APPEARANCE

If you've been to a nursing home lately, you know that it can be a pretty scary sight. You probably saw a bunch of women (because they're more likely to survive their spouses) sitting in a row, nodding their heads, smiling vacantly, or calling to people who aren't there.

As we age, we can become terrified that we're going to lose our sight, our memory, our mobility, our independence, our friends, and even our homes. But it doesn't have to be this way! We can start remodeling our bodily houses with the tools in this chapter.

Loving the Skin You're In

Thanks to our diet, lifestyle, and environment—along with thousands of years of evolution—we've currently arrived at the point in our history when we're living longer than humans ever have. But are we living any *better?*

The reason I wrote this book is so that it could be an important resource for everyone, not just a "light dusting" filled with some airy-fairy notions about aging. Along with that, I know that the way we look is central to our self-esteem and maybe even our jobs. In speaking with my Los Angeles clients, I was taken aback when I found out that their very livelihoods could be in jeopardy as a result of revealing their age.

Why is it that a mature man looks handsome and distinguished whereas a similarly aged woman just looks old? As a well-known Manhattan hairdresser once said, "There's a lot of pain in not being beautiful." It can be very difficult to bear witness to the ravages of time, which it seems we're powerless to stop. What can we do when the 49th parallel moves 20 degrees farther south? I'm not beautiful, but I do think I'm attractive, so what must a real beauty feel when she looks in the mirror as the years go by? Is this what happened to the legendary Greta Garbo, who rarely showed her face to the public once she reached a certain age?

I'm more impressed by stories of women who don't let their age send them into hiding, such as the iconic sex symbol Brigitte Bardot, who parlayed her beauty and fame into animal activism; or Tina Turner, the famous pop singer who continues to perform and is going strong well into her 60s. Tina still looks fabulous, but she's also physically active and enjoys a very healthy way of life on the edge of the Mediterranean in the south of France.

Of course Tina is also African American, and non-Caucasians tend to have much thicker, sturdier skin than Caucasians do. Many times, it can be difficult to tell the age of Hispanics, Polynesians, or African Americans because they often have a lot more moisture and natural oils in their skin and generally wear their age well. (Yet while they may look youthful on the outside, they have just as many age-related issues on the inside as everyone else does.)

When collagen starts to break down, Caucasian people appear to age more quickly. I don't know that my skin ever had a chance, as I was born in Scotland, the land of light-skinned people. My family can be traced back to the 12th century, and before that we were probably descended from the Norse of Scandinavia. On top of all that, I compounded my hereditary skin-related issues by years of suntanning in my youth.

I remember in particular the summer between the 11th and 12th grades, when I went to visit my parents in India. Every day after lunch, my sister and I would go up to the rooftop garden to smoke French cigarettes and bake in the sun. I tanned for years and greatly enjoyed it, never realizing the price I'd have to pay later on. Today, I have delicate, weathered skin.

While I was baking in the heat of the noonday sun, my friend Judy, on the other hand, was reading a book in the shade and wearing a large straw hat. Now in her 60s, she is reaping the rewards and has lovely, milky white skin.

My sister, who is four years younger than I am, has beautiful hands. She's preserved them well, wearing rubber gloves while gardening or to do any cleaning, and her hands never touch dishwater. She was thinking ahead. Contrast this with my hands, which are weathered from washing dishes, swimming in the ocean, painting walls and pictures, kneading bread (in the old days), gardening, building furniture, and caring for children. I'm truly a hands-on person.

Now that I'm in my 60s, I realize the importance of taking care of my hands. I take silica capsules, which come from the herb horsetail. (Hair, nails, and skin contain silica, which becomes depleted with age.) I also take buckwheat-seed tablets to strengthen skin cells and repair broken capillaries. In addition, I drink lots of water, eat fish frequently, use olive oil, and take fish oils daily in capsule form. I use a wonderful hand cream from the French company L'Occitane that's rich and moisturizing. And, of course, I no longer bake in the sun.

The sun isn't the only culprit that can weaken and weather the skin—chemicals can, too. Any substance that you put on your skin is absorbed directly into your bloodstream. Thus, with daily applications of skin-care products, you may be soaking up potential toxins without filtering of any kind. Know that almost all of the big-name skin-care lines use some sort of toxic ingredients.

Take a look at the products you use and make sure that they're natural and chemical free. Any product that contains parabens, sodium laurel sulphate, or anything else you don't recognize should be avoided. Hundreds of new chemicals and preservatives are released into the marketplace each year; fortunately, we're becoming more aware of the toxic-chemical issue, and there are more natural cosmetics available today than ever before.

I use an herbal non-soap cleanser, a skin-care line from Europe, and the rest of the work I do is on the inside. I avoid foods that wrinkle and thin the skin, such as coffee; alcohol; sugar; processed, white-flour products like bread and pasta; and additives and preservatives.

The very best way to have great skin is to change your diet. Skin is the last manifestation of the gut, so if you want a great complexion, eat healthfully! I recommend that you check out *The Perricone Prescription: A Physician's 28-Day Program for Total Body and Face Rejuvenation,* by Dr. Nicholas Perricone, as his philosophy and nutritional guidelines promote great skin.

⁓

Aging is about reviewing our history, pampering ourselves, and maintaining what we have—as the years tick by, we want to look as good as we can while becoming proud legends. There's a story behind every gray hair and a wealth of experience in each wrinkle. However, growing old does have its challenges, and I believe that Sandie's voice speaks for millions of us:

> I've been fortunate to be what this society considers beautiful, and I've become so used to turning heads whenever I walk into a room. I think it's going to be harder for me to grow old because the heads aren't turning as much now. I'm 48 years old and still look like I'm in my 30s, and I was blessed with a body that has aged well. Yet I know that's not going to last forever, so it does scare me.
>
> I think it's difficult for someone who's been told that she's beautiful most of her life to go through the transition from what's considered beautiful to appearing old. But then I look at women in their 60s who are still stunning—they're healthy; vibrant; and, yes, beautiful—and it gives me hope and strength.
>
> I realize that I'm going to get old and have some wrinkles no matter what, but true beauty comes from within. Of course I want to be healthy as I get older,

but I have to admit that coming to terms with looking old was actually my biggest challenge.

Now that I've been around for a while, I've had a few people in my life pass away, and it's really strange to think that one day they're here, and the next, they're gone. I really don't think about dying much, because I'm too busy wondering if I'm *living* enough. I do need to stop saying the word *should* and just accept that I'm doing the best I can today—I'm grateful to wake up each morning and have another chance to enjoy the wonderful life I've been given.

Aging Skin

"Where are you going, my pretty maid?" goes the nursery rhyme. "I'm going a-milking, sir," the young lady says. When asked, "What is your fortune, my pretty maid?" she responds, "My face is my fortune, sir." Fortune or no fortune, here's the skinny on what happens to our skin as we age.

When we were in our mid-30s, most of us retained the fresh, smooth skin of our youth, with nary a wrinkle to be seen. At that age, because skin and facial muscles were still firm and elastic, our contours remained smooth and well defined. Around the age of 35, we may remember the odd gray hair or a wrinkle or two appearing. The aging process happens so gradually that many of us didn't even notice it until we looked back through our photo albums and saw the difference ten or even five years made.

The first signs of aging appear when our upper-cheek muscles start to collapse. By the age of 45, as estrogen levels decline, these muscles can elongate by as much as half an inch, dragging the skin over the cheeks and downward to form those plump little jowls on either side of our mouths.

At the same time that our cheeks are collapsing toward the South Pole, the muscles under our chins become looser, and the jawline loses its shape. Next the eyes start to go: Tiny muscles stretch and can cause the outer corners of the upper eyelids to droop over the lower lids. Now our alert, fresh look of youth disappears. These heavy eyelids contain many lines and folds, and our makeup smears, our vision might be affected, and we can develop bags under the eyes.

The process continues, and by the age of 55, the upper-cheek muscles continue to stretch by at least three-quarters of an inch, forming more creases around the ears, mouth, and jawline. Neck muscles lose their tone, become slack, and start to form horizontal lines and rolls or cords. Then the loose, stretched skin sags downward toward the front of the neck—the tip of our chin looks like an extension of our neck, and the next demoralizing turn of events is the "turkey neck" of old age. The bottom line is that with time, our skin actually falls off our face!

It's no wonder that beating back the hands of Father Time is big business. Thousands of men and women are actively seeking cosmetic treatments and are willing to pay whatever it takes. For them, the aging process is denied for as long as possible.

Exploring the Options

Every year in Las Vegas and several other cities around the world, there are annual conferences on aging held by the group A4M, the American Academy of Anti-Aging Medicine. These are exciting, leading-edge expositions devoted to longevity strategies, techniques, procedures, and products geared toward the aging population. As part of my book research, I attended one of these conferences last year and heard several presentations on bio-identical hormone balancing, stem-cell therapies, brain-function enhancement, and nutritional approaches.

A4M attracts many dedicated doctors and health professionals from all over the world who know that anti-aging medicine is the wave of the future, and they gather to share breakthroughs in preventing and treating diseases related to the biological process of aging. Many of the professionals involved in longevity medicine believe, as far-fetched as it seems, that by the year 2050 the average healthy human will be able to live to 150 years of age. (Please visit: **www.A4M.com**.)

At these conferences, you'll also hear presentations about various procedures such as plastic surgery (including face-lifts); Botox, facial fillers, chemical peels, and other nonsurgical cosmetic practices; as well as skin treatments and skin-care products. All of these are designed to ward off the ravages of time for a few more years.

This book wouldn't be complete without at least some discussion of the various skin-treatment options currently available, especially since I called this book *The Body Knows . . . How to Stay Young*. Part of staying youthful and optimistic involves appearance because when you look good, you feel good. But regardless of whatever treatments you use on your skin, what really matters is the condition of your *insides*. Organ function and attitude are the real determining factors of your age.

Unfortunately, thanks to the fashion and entertainment industries, we in Western cultures celebrate a youth that is largely concerned with only one thing: appearance. The mature or elderly person is undervalued, discredited, and disdained. To the young, aging is simply not accepted as a "cool" thing to be doing. This has spawned a highly lucrative cosmetic-procedures industry.

I have two skin specialists: one is a dermatologist, and the other is a plastic surgeon. My dermatologist looks over my entire body every year for suspicious-looking moles and potential skin cancers or spots caused by sun damage. My plastic surgeon has performed a delicate operation to repair severed nerves and tendons after I accidentally jabbed a knife into my ring finger while removing an avocado pit. Both of these doctors are very busy and no doubt very wealthy. Thanks to all the baby boomers now reaching their 60s and beyond, I don't think that their practices will do anything but continue to flourish.

I actually had my first encounter with plastic surgery at the age of 22. I had huge breasts, long before the days of the legendary chests of Dolly Parton or Pamela Anderson. Mine was the era of Audrey Hepburn, when small breasts were barely noticeable under a cashmere sweater and a string of pearls.

At 15 years of age, I weighed 108 pounds and hardly needed a bra. By the time I turned 18—after having spent almost two years at a boarding school in Switzerland and living on kilos of cheese, baguettes, and chocolate—I weighed 140 pounds. My breasts were the size of melons, and buying bras and bathing suits was a problem. As my maiden aunt's breasts started underneath her chin and ended up just above her waistline, and my mother was full breasted, it looked like I'd inherited the family trait, too.

Men never looked at me as a whole, but they sure went gaga over my breasts; I was miserable, uncomfortable, and embarrassed. Finally, it became time to do something about it, and I went under the knife a few days after my 22nd birthday. Five pounds of breast tissue were removed (imagine five pounds of butter lined up on your kitchen counter!), and I was returned to a size-34 brassiere. My self-esteem went through the roof, and I've never looked back.

I can attest that any surgical procedure that enhances the way a person feels about him- or herself is an important one. But when it comes to radical surgeries that counteract the effects of aging, do be sure to weigh the pros and cons carefully.

Noninvasive Procedures

Facial lines and wrinkles are caused by the thinning of the collagen layer under the skin, and regardless of what all the beauty-product companies tell you, topical creams cannot diminish the lines and wrinkles caused by collagen loss.

So now I'd like to go over some of the noninvasive skin treatments that are currently available to "freshen" aging skin (and please keep in mind that risks can be involved with them, so only allow yourself to be treated by a reputable practitioner):

1. Thermage. I asked my dermatologist about the latest procedure that she felt was the most effective and popular for aging women. She didn't hesitate to recommend Thermage, a new treatment where loose skin can be treated with nonsurgical technology. It works by heating a large volume of collagen in the deeper layers of the skin and its underlying tissue, while simultaneously protecting the outer layer of skin with cooling. The Thermage procedure stimulates collagen production and lifts and tightens sagging skin, all without surgery or recovery time.

2. **Botox** is now the most commonly performed cosmetic procedure in the United States. The treatment involves the injection of a tiny amount of botulinum toxin, which relaxes select muscles and limits their ability to contract and form lines. After treatment, the skin lies flat and unwrinkled, while the rest of the facial muscles contract in their normal fashion, thus not affecting overall facial expression. The most popular area of the face for Botox treatments is between the brows or the crow's-feet area at the edge of the eye.

Women aren't the only ones seeking age-enhancing treatments—vast numbers of men are doing so, too. To that end, last year I interviewed Dr. Eric Kaplan on my radio show. Kaplan is a chiropractor in Florida, the anti-aging capital of the U.S., and he too lined up for Botox treatments. However, he inadvertently received pure botulinum toxin, which severely affected his nervous system. Subsequently, Eric and his wife, who also had Botox treatments, spent two years in rehabilitation learning to talk, walk, eat, and speak. His book *Dying to Be Young: From Botox to Botulism—A True Story of Survival* (Nightengale Press) documents this unfortunate saga. So know your practitioner and your treatments, and be aware of all potential side effects.

3. Collagen replacement reminds me of actress Goldie Hawn in the movie *The First Wives Club*. In one of the first scenes, we see a "blubber mouthed" Goldie (not the way she usually looks) receiving yet another injection to plump up her lips, and it's not a pretty sight.

Collagen is an injectable filling agent, and it remains the most popular product for skin and soft-tissue augmentation. It's considered a nonsurgical procedure that smooths out facial lines and plumps up wrinkles and scars by replenishing the natural collagen under the skin.

4. Chemical peels. It's surprising what people will do to feel loved. Take Margaret, for example, who started dating Chris when she was 52 and he was 45. Even though there was a significant age gap, they both seemed very happy in each other's company. Nevertheless, three years into the relationship, Margaret kept seeing the effects of gravity whenever she caught sight of her reflection, and she continually felt the pressure of her compounding years. Would Chris still love her as she looked older? To assuage these concerns, she got a chemical peel.

I understand that chemical-peel products have changed and improved over the years, but Margaret dove into the fray more than 20 years ago. She spent a good two weeks under wraps and behind closed doors until the procedure healed. Sadly, her facial tissue didn't respond favorably to the peel, so scar tissue began to build up. Because her top layer of skin had peeled off thanks to the chemicals, her skin lost its pigment, and she constantly had to cover it up with makeup. She looked awful, which didn't help her self-esteem. Every time she looked at herself in the mirror, she wondered why she'd made the decision to try to alter the course of time. But she and Chris continued to do things together and even planned an around-the-world sailing trip.

Six weeks into their voyage, the couple ran into bad weather off the coast of California. They started fighting, and every emotion rose to the surface. They ended up parting company on the dock in Long Beach, and Margaret packed her bags and took the bus back to her home in Seattle. She felt bereft, lost, and alone; and her self-esteem was at its lowest ebb. She realized that her personal worth and value were based on what others like Chris thought of her, and she was willing to put herself through a personally disastrous procedure with permanent consequences all in the name of love and acceptance. Her next step was to put her life back together by learning to love herself and her body, regardless of how she looked.

5. Laser skin rejuvenation. I was introduced to laser therapy in 2005. I didn't choose it for myself, but it was my dermatologist's treatment of choice for removing several actinic keratosis lesions on my upper lip, the result of many years spent baking in the sun.

Laser skin resurfacing is a safe process that uses an infrared light to tighten skin and reverse the signs of aging; it's designed to stimulate long-term collagen rebuilding, thus creating younger-looking skin. In my experience, there's little pain during the procedure, but there's significant pain afterward. My dermatologist only treated a small portion of the skin on my upper lip, but the discomfort, burning, and crusting (not to mention having to be secluded for more than a week) was not fun. I felt as if I'd been burned by napalm, and I seriously doubted my dermatologist's wisdom.

Yet this period of being cooped up gave me time to write *The Body "Knows" Cookbook,* so I managed to make the experience useful. The treatment did turn out to be successful—I haven't had a return of sun damage on my upper lip, and the skin in that area has returned to its youthful appearance.

6. Photorejuvenation. Over time, many men and women develop age spots on their hands as a result of a poorly functioning liver, low sugar metabolism, and sun damage. This brings us to Carla, an antiques dealer who lives in the glamorous and fascinating world of Christie's and Sotheby's auction houses in New York and London. She attends sales in castles in Germany and estates in France, and her hands are always on view. Thus, she was a perfect candidate for an interesting new therapy to remove age spots.

Photorejuvenation is another "miracle technology" designed to stimulate collagen production and plump up aging skin. Because red blemishes from broken blood vessels and brown spots of pigment from sun damage respond to intense pulsed light, such light is passed over the backs of the hands at about one-inch intervals. As Carla described it, "It felt like a rubber band snapping back and hitting me on the hand every time the light was pulsed. There was a little 'ouch' feeling."

Since Carla's hands were heated, there was a burning sensation for a few days, and she had to keep her hands out of water (especially hot water). But after that, all of her age spots turned a very dark brown, and then they crusted over and dropped off. Today, the backs of her hands are much healthier, revealing a mere hint of the age spots.

7. Facial-toning equipment. There are many ways to skin a cat, not to mention a human face. There are treatments that don't involve cutting, burning, peeling, or injecting, which are less expensive and less extreme options. Because muscle tone supports your skin, facial-toning equipment—which uses mild electrical stimulation to activate cells and retrain muscles—might provide an answer for you.

It's a known fact that low-level currents have a healing effect, and this is explained in *The Body Electric: Electromagnetism and the Foundation of Life,* by Robert O. Becker, M.D., and Gary Selden (Morrow). In this fascinating book, Dr. Becker offers important clues to the healing process in the long-discarded theory that electricity is vital to life. His discoveries point to a day when human organs, limbs, and spinal cords may be able to regenerate by using electrical currents.

Most physical therapists use low-level, frequency-generating equipment such as TENS machines to help heal injuries. These machines deliver small electrical pulses to the body through electrodes that are placed on the skin. The pulses block nerve-pain pathways to the brain, increase blood supply to the area where the electrodes are placed, and stimulate the body's own pain-easing chemicals called "endorphins."

Similarly, facial-toning equipment uses low frequencies that can't be felt in order to tighten and tone, reduce puffiness, and soften wrinkles. My neighbor Helena, for instance, is in her mid-50s and has beautiful tight skin. She owns her own facial-toning machine and uses it twice a week, and I'm certainly impressed by how she looks.

Likewise, Cathi Watson, a renowned Chicago radio personality, swears by her facial-toning machine, which she also uses twice a week. She's dedicated to doing her facial-toning exercises every day as well (see below). Now in her 70s, Cathi's skin is tight and youthful. (Please visit: **www.ageless4life.com**.)

Prices for facial-toning equipment vary from $2,000 to $4,000 per unit or less. I happen to like a handheld unit that sells for about $300.

8. Facial-toning exercises. Donna, 65, and Fred, 71, have been doing facial-toning exercises for the past two decades. They were shown the method years ago by an Austrian cosmetician who told Donna and Fred that if they spent five minutes doing them every day, this would prevent sagging facial skin. So they've been stretching out their tongues to reach their noses, pulling their mouths up to the left and then the right, and scrunching their eyes in the process—but they both look pretty good. (However, I did notice that there was a brochure for facial fillers on Donna's kitchen counter when I last visited for dinner.)

Donna taught me the exercises, which I faithfully do while driving. Here's how:

- Stretch your tongue out as far as you can. Now curl it up and try to reach for your nose and hold it there for as long as you can— optimally five minutes. (I count road signs— I say to myself that I will hold this position until I drive to the next road sign.) You'll notice that this exercise tightens the muscles in your chin and your neck.

• Take your lower jaw and move it out until it juts out beyond your upper jaw. Hold that position for up to five minutes. You'll notice that this tightens your entire chin and lower-jaw area.

• Put your upper lip into a sneer. Take the sneer up to the right and scrunch your right eye in the process. Hold that pose for five minutes. Repeat the previous step but on the left side of your face. You'll notice that this tightens the muscles in your cheek.

• With your teeth held together, open your lips and say "E." Continue to open your lips until you can feel your cheeks tightening and your neck muscles pronounced, tight and firm. Hold this position for five minutes.

Look on the Internet for other facial-toning exercises.

Meeting Fatima

In the middle of researching skin-enhancing techniques, I received a knock on my door and met Fatima. A friend had suggested that she come to me for a reading, but it turned out that *I* would be the one receiving the gift.

Fatima was born in Iran, formerly Persia. When she was eight years old, her grandmother taught her an ancient beauty technique for firming the skin that would change her life—a secret not found in any book. Fatima's grandmother was the personal beautician to a wealthy family closely connected to the Shah of Iran. Women at the family compound (just like many women all over the world) were very focused on their looks and would do anything to be trim and beautiful. Beauty treatments and preparations would be given to these women on a weekly basis . . . it was a priority.

Natural masks of yogurt and lemon or egg white were applied to the face of the regal mistress of the house to keep her beautiful and happy. And one of the special treatments she received was a delicate procedure using fine thread passed over the skin as an efficient exfoliating technique. Called a "thread face-lift," this technique is also used in India as a way to remove hair from the face, but Fatima's grandmother used it to stimulate the growth of new skin cells, with remarkable results.

Every week Fatima was taught how to perform this procedure on her grandmother, who told her that it would give Fatima youthful and beautiful skin for the rest of her life. Finally, after eight years of training, her grandmother deemed Fatima to be proficient and sent her out into the world to use the thread-lift technique on other women.

Although Fatima is now 52 years old, she still has tight, plump skin as a result of this procedure—and the day she knocked on my door, I experienced the treatment for myself. As she stood before me with her yards of twisted thread, I knew I was being visited by a master.

She worked on my face with quick, deft movements, explaining, "You have millions of skin cells, and they need to be stimulated. The skin rarely receives the stimulation that other parts of the body get. It is the stimulation of the skin in this manner that encourages the growth of new skin cells, elasticity, and collagen production. Healthy skin creates its own natural moisture."

Evidently, as the twisted thread is passed over the face in subtle and delicate movements, it grabs tiny sections of skin, which are lifted and stimulated. This draws the blood to the surface of the skin to rejuvenate it.

For me, the procedure felt like a butterfly's wing passing over my skin, lifting and stimulating it. I was in heaven! After about 15 minutes, Fatima was done, and every part of my face and neck tingled. She suggested that the procedure be done once a week for eight weeks, then maintenance should be scheduled every two to three weeks. (Please visit: **www.fatimasnaturalfacelift. com.**)

Fatima has loyal clients who come from all around to see her, and while she works on their faces, she serves them mint tea, a traditional beverage in Iran. She kindly shared her recipe with me, which can be found on page 287.

Radiating Energy

Have you ever thought of radiating energy? You see, since energy heals, when it's radiated to a specific area of the body, it can have a rejuvenating effect.

You can use a healing frequency on your own skin by rubbing your hands together and placing them on your face. Send the resonating frequency of love and healing there as you also "tone" a note that feels right to you. Just hum that note quietly to yourself under your breath; after doing so for a few minutes, you'll be able to feel your face tingle as if the cells are vibrating. And you can visualize a color beaming into your face—such as a soft pink, an effervescent peach, or a golden bronze—which adds an additional healing dimension to your skin's radiance.

Here's another simple exercise that will bring you instant radiance:

1. Close your eyes and breathe deeply and rhythmically, in and out.

2. Focus on the skin on your face, and start to pour loving energy into it.

3. Now choose a word from the following selection:

    *   *Excitement*
    *   *Happiness*
    *   *Joy*
    *   *Zest*
    *   *Success*
    *   *Energy*

    Breathe the word that feels right for you into your skin—in and out. (I like the word *excitement*.) Note how excited or happy you feel when you repeat this word over and over in your mind, and understand that that quality is being translated into your skin.

4. There are other words that you can use for other purposes as well. Here are some examples:

- *Peace*
- *Rest*
- *Tranquil*
- *Calm*
- *Stable*

Close your eyes and say to yourself whichever word you prefer, paying attention to where you feel the vibration or energy in your body.

This exercise in "heart words" illustrates how positive feelings bring good things into your life. So when you think about your desire to have youthful skin, realize that you're actually wishing to feel youthful in all aspects of your life. When you feel good, you look good. And feelings can't be bought, because they're manufactured by you!

Simple Beauty Strategies

Many years ago I was involved in the fashion industry (I even had my own weekly newspaper column), and one of the most enjoyable aspects of my work was organizing makeovers for men and women. I learned lots of little tricks to make people look younger and more vital, and I'd like to share a few of them with you.

Here are some suggestions for easily maximizing your beauty potential:

1. Take Care of Your Teeth

While teeth whitening wasn't done during my fashion makeovers, it's still important to consider. Teeth enamel wears away over the years, revealing the softer and darker layer underneath; teeth also become yellow or discolored due to staining from coffee, nicotine, and various foods. Teeth whitening can take years off your age and give you a great smile.

Several years ago, this process was done in a dentist's office at great expense, as impressions had to be taken of the upper and lower teeth, and special trays had to be made to hold the whitening gel. Nowadays, whitening strips are available at your local drugstore. A strip is applied to the upper and lower teeth, held in place for about 20 minutes, and your teeth are instantly whiter. Yet due to the chemicals in the strips, it's advised that you don't use them too frequently. My dental hygienist recommends that teeth whiteners should only be used every six months. She told me that teeth-whitening toothpaste is fine, and if you eliminate coffee and black tea, you'll notice that you have less staining.

As we age, we need to preserve our teeth. Thanks to my parents being sticklers about oral hygiene when I was growing up, I only have six fillings in my mouth. Then about 25 years ago, I had all of my black mercury-amalgam fillings removed and replaced with gold or composite. This is something that you should consider doing as well, for you may not know that each tooth sits on an energy line or meridian and is linked to an organ or system. A leaking mercury-amalgam filling can be affecting a part of your body that you're not even aware of, so meet with your dentist and create a plan to have those fillings replaced.

Gum disease and loose teeth are the result of poor dental hygiene and nutrition. Bob came to me because several of his teeth were becoming loose, pointing to a B-vitamin deficiency. A beneficial way to assimilate iron and B vitamins is to eat red meat, the subject of much negative press. Bob had indeed stopped eating it because he'd heard that it was bad for his heart, but I let him know that red meat and B vitamins support the electrical impulses of the heart, and iron and B vitamins are important for cell repair. Bob began eating red meat twice a week, and within several weeks, his teeth were more solid in his jaw.

2. Use Color to Enhance Your Eyes

It's said that the eyes are the windows to the soul. Since we've already discussed improving the eyes from a nutritional level, let's discuss them from a purely cosmetic point of view.

Look in the mirror and deeply observe the color of your eyes. Next, choose about ten articles of clothing in different hues and hold them up to your face. Notice which colors enhance your eyes and make them stand out—these are the ones that are best for you to wear by your face.

As we age, skin tone and pigmentation tend to become dull, and we actually lose the natural skin color associated with our youth. Choosing soft colors for clothing can lift the radiance of our skin and make it appear to have more color tone.

My former mother-in-law really knew her colors, and she was a striking woman with silver hair and a ruddy complexion that she never covered up with cosmetics. Her best color was blue, which emphasized her eyes and her hair.

I also find that when women wear brighter lipstick, it tends to emphasize the eyes, which seem to "pop" out. But stay away from really bright lipstick, such as neon pink and bright red, as these colors can make you look older and are in direct contrast to aging skin. Also, try to avoid using lipsticks with a dark brown tone, since they can make you look like a cadaver. (I prefer corals and pinks.) In addition, cheek blush and a terra-cotta bronzer can enhance the color of your eyes.

It's a good idea to have a consultation with any of the cosmetologists in department or makeup stores to get some ideas. This will give you a chance to see what's available, test out colors, and get a sense of what's right for you. Do be sure that you only buy organic and chemical-free makeup, however.

3. Don't Forget Your Hair

Always use a good-quality shampoo. And here's a great tip for healthy hair: Add two tablespoons of coconut oil, which nourishes the skin and hair, to your daily diet. Women in India have used this trick for centuries.

As for color, I started pulling gray hairs out of my head at age 35 . . . then I realized that there were too many to pull. I dyed my hair the medium brown of my youth, which did not look flattering. So I had a consultation with a wonderful hairstylist who had just arrived from London, and he recommended that I look into highlights. Because I have a fair complexion, the dark dye made me look as if I had a hat on my head—it was far too overpowering. The blonde-and-gold highlights that he suggested covered the gray and enhanced the color of my skin.

Once in a while I think about letting my hair go salt and pepper; but then I feel too young for that, so I've opted to continue to streak my hair. My hairdresser does it so that the chemicals aren't applied directly to my scalp. Ask for chemical-free hair color, now available in some salons. Remember, chemicals that are absorbed directly into the skin end up in the body. Any kind of chemical exposure warrants doing some sort of liver detoxification on a daily basis, so ask someone at the health-food store for a supplement for this purpose.

Since I've learned about nutritional arterial cleansing (oral chelation) and balancing hormones, my hair is beginning to return to its natural color. I look forward to this continuing.

Whenever I see women I admire who are in their 80s and 90s, I find that those who look their best have some sort of beauty regimen in which styling their hair is a big part. So my advice is that you consult a good hairdresser and get some ideas about what would be most attractive for you. By tuning in to your individual style and then bringing it out, you'll come alive.

Healing the Eyes

It can be pretty scary when vision declines. Earlier in the book I explained the relationship of liver detoxification to eyesight, so you know the importance of working on your body and correcting your nutrition in protecting your eyes. This section will delve into the subject more deeply.

Macular degeneration is the most common cause of blindness in people over the age of 55 and is usually found in elderly adults. This is a condition in which the center of the inner lining of the eye, known as the "macula" area of the retina, suffers thinning, atrophy, and even bleeding in some cases. The result can be the loss of central vision, along with the inability to see details, to read, or even to recognize faces.

Many years ago I was introduced to the work of Dr. Edward C. Kondrot, M.D., author of *Healing the Eye the Natural Way: Alternative Medicine and Macular Degeneration* (North Atlantic Books). An ophthalmologist and homeopath in Phoenix, Dr. Kondrot discusses methods of correcting macular degeneration in this book and on his Website: **www.healingtheeye.com.**

When treating macular degeneration and diseases of the eye, Dr. Kondrot implements several strategies: diet; specific supplementation; microcurrent therapy; and intravenous chelation, which is an innovative therapy involving the use of a synthetic amino acid (EDTA) that binds to calcium, lead, cadmium, mercury, and trace minerals. These minerals are fed into the vein, and after combining with the EDTA, they're eliminated from the body through the kidneys into the urine.

For many years, chelation therapy has been used for patients with heavy-metal toxicity or poor circulation due to plaque buildup in the arteries (called "arteriosclerosis"). It's believed that the causes of macular degeneration include arteriosclerosis, toxicity, and cell damage. During the intravenous chelation process, arterial plaque is slowly dissolved, thus improving blood flow throughout the body—and targeting healing to the eyes.

Chelation doesn't have to be done intravenously; in fact, many people respond well to oral chelation (pills taken by mouth). I think that oral chelation and vascular cleansing are both very useful for overall health.

Along with intravenous chelation, Dr. Kondrot's patients who suffer from macular degeneration are given a change in diet and specific supplementation, as well as microcurrent therapy, which is applied to the outside of the eye. Here, a tiny current stimulates and encourages blood supply to the area, thus improving the function of retinal cells.

Three years ago, Graham was diagnosed with macular degeneration, but as a result of following Dr. Kondrot's protocol, he's back to driving and playing golf. Then there's Gladys, who's been dealing with macular degeneration for 15 years. We've talked about her situation, and despite my suggestions to explore alternative therapies such as those suggested by Dr. Kondrot, she's of the old school. Good vision depends on a good diet, yet she protested, "Caroline, how could I give up my morning cups of coffee, or my cinnamon rolls and chocolate? These give me so much pleasure."

Gladys has reason to need pleasure and comfort in her life. In the past year, her husband, Louis, has been diagnosed with Alzheimer's disease, and if the disease continues to progress, he'll be placed in a long-term-care facility. After many years of marriage, Gladys's personal vision of what she sees for her life has been derailed, and nothing is going to happen for her physically unless she changes emotionally and spiritually.

Eye Exercises

You can improve your vision by exercising your eyes. Brain Gym offers a set of exercises designed to stimulate vision, memory, reading, and coordination; over the years, I've seen marvelous results thanks to their exercises. Their Website (**www.braingym.org**) offers books, tapes, and CDs regarding specific physical activities that have been shown to enhance concentration and cognitive and learning abilities. The exercises that follow are just three examples of what Brain Gym offers.

1. Here's one called "Lazy Eights":

- Take your right arm and stretch it out in front of you. Loosely close your hand and place your thumb directly up.

- Now make a wide figure eight in the air, without bending your arm. Keep your eyes focused on your thumb.

- Continue to create about ten figure eights, all the while saying, "I can see my future—my vision is clear."

- Now change to your left arm, keeping your eyes clearly focused on your thumb, and repeat your affirmation.

- Repeat this exercise several times a day.

2. Here's another great eye-strengthening exercise:

- Again, stretch your arm out and point your thumb upward.

- Focus your eyes on your thumb and draw it very closely back toward your face.

- Keeping your eyes on your thumb, very slowly stretch your arm back out again.

- Do this sequence five times.

3. This is called the "healing hands" exercise, and it's best done while lying down:

- Rub your hands together to generate energy and warmth.

- Close your eyes, cup your hands, and place your palms over your eyes, keeping in mind that there is healing power in the hands.

- Radiate this energy to your eyes for about five minutes. At the same time, say to yourself, "My eyes rest and regenerate."

Another unusual way to improve your eyesight is to purchase a pair of "pinhole glasses" and wear them for about half an hour each day. These are sunglasses that have many little holes in the lenses, the purpose of which is to focus your vision "through" them, thus strengthening or exercising your eyes.

I was introduced to pinhole glasses by a friend in Sacramento, but they have quite a history, dating back to ancient China. I wear mine often and notice that my vision is definitely sharper after using them. There are many sources for these glasses on the Internet, and you don't need anything fancy—just the regular ones that cost about $20.

Repairing Nerves and Regaining Balance

Do you remember a time in your youth when you could scamper down a flight of stairs without holding on to the handrail, or hop over obstacles and land firmly on your feet with perfect balance?

Try this experiment: While holding on to the back of a chair, close your eyes and stand on one foot. Now let go of the chair—can you balance on one leg with your eyes closed? If so, your balance is good. If not, there is work to be done.

Over and over again I see people who are overstimulated and unstable on their feet. At the risk of sounding repetitious, overstimulation is a result of too little protein and too much caffeine, sugar, or starch. A great example of this comes from Leo, who suffers from Parkinson's disease. When I went with friends to visit him, I knew that overstimulation was part of his problem.

When I asked him about his diet, he sheepishly took a large plastic box out of the cupboard; it was filled with a well-known brand of dark-chocolate bars, in the extra-large size. Each day Leo would eat a whole bar—this amount of stimulation from chocolate on a daily basis was not helping his condition, particularly since he was a fragile person of Finnish descent.

Protein is calming and can help balance blood sugars, thus affecting balance. I suggest small, frequent meals that contain from one to four ounces of protein. If you find that you're edgy, jittery, or off balance, eliminate your morning java or black tea and add a few ounces of protein with meals (especially breakfast). Using digestive enzymes as part of your supplementation regimen will ensure that your proteins are being absorbed. And supplementing with the hormone testosterone can really help with balance and focus.

Also, stand tall and hold your head up. Whenever I see a hunched-over elderly person, this prompts me to recall my ballet classes and focus on my posture. Now, while in my youth I could scramble over logs on the beach, climb trees, and ride my bicycle with perfect balance, I no longer take these kinds of chances. My balance is good, but I *am* 64—so I look where I'm walking and keep my focus. Since I'm an entrepreneur, an injury would greatly hamper my lifestyle.

Great ways to repair nerves are: getting a good night's sleep, making sure that there's consistent protein in the diet, eliminating stimulants, balancing hormones, meditating daily, and practicing balance exercises.

Following are the balance exercises that I find most useful (be sure to use the back of a chair for stability):

1. Stand tall and keep your back straight. With your left hand on the chair's back, lift your right foot and place it at a right angle to your knee. Hold this pose and focus your eyes on a spot on the wall, or look through the window and focus on a tree, plant, or item in nature. Hold your focus; when you feel balanced in this position, take your hand off the chair. Put your hands together and place them in a prayer position over your heart. Hold the prayer pose for several minutes while breathing deeply. Then switch positions and repeat the exercise using your left foot.

2. Stand tall and keep your back straight. With your right hand on the chair's back, slowly lean forward and stretch out your left leg behind you. Keep your leg straight and your tummy muscles tight, and breathe deeply. With your left hand pointing forward, level with your nose, point your fingers straight ahead. Focus your fingers and your eyes on a spot on the wall or outside. When you feel balanced, take your right hand off the chair. Reach forward and place it beside your left hand, which is still pointing forward. Keep your focus, keep your tummy muscles tight, and breathe deeply. Hold this pose for as long as you feel comfortable. Switch legs.

3. Stand tall and keep your back straight. With your left hand on the chair's back, place your right hand out to the side at shoulder height. Lift your right leg out in front of you and up as high as you can. Keeping the leg straight, point your toes and hold that position. Remember to breathe. When you feel balanced, let go of the chair and put your left hand out to the side at shoulder height. Focus on a spot on the wall or outside, and hold

that position for as long as you feel comfortable. Repeat this exercise with your left leg.

Exercise Keeps Us Young

I'm sure you know that exercise is important, but how dedicated are you to it? If you don't feel like exercising, I can almost guarantee that when you follow the guidelines for removing addictions, toxins, and allergens from your body, the energy and desire to exercise will naturally come to the surface. When the body is healthy and full of energy, it just wants to move. This will be the case for you, too—your body will propel you out the door with almost no choice from you in the matter. Then what used to be a chore becomes a pleasure.

If you're complaining of hip, knee, and joint pain, here's a story for you. After being a distance runner in his 40s and 50s, Doug was considering having his knee joints replaced due to severe arthritis. When it was discovered that he was allergic to every food that he was eating, he went through a period of food avoidance and nutritional supplementation, and the pain in his knees was alleviated. Doug was able to avoid an expensive and painful surgery. His exercise has changed completely, and now he does strength-training and water exercises three times a week.

Then there are Maureen and Ralph, who are in their 70s. They've always been very active, but they hadn't had a consistent workout routine until Maureen was diagnosed with osteoporosis, and her doctor ordered weight-bearing exercise. For the past few months, Maureen and Ralph have worked with a trainer at the gym, lifting light weights and using specific equipment that tones muscles without damage or strain. Maureen reports that she's never felt better in her life.

Exercise oxygenates the cells, gives us energy, controls hunger, and helps create an optimistic outlook. Yet I love what cardiologist Al Sears says: Contrary to what we've been told, it's not true that working out 30 to 60 minutes, three or four times a week, is necessary for cardiovascular health . . . and it may even be damaging.

Dr. Sears gives an encouraging option of reconditioning your heart and lungs with as little as ten minutes of cardiovascular exercise a day. He suggests short burst of exercise with periods of rest in between. Over a period of weeks and months, these short burst of exercise gradually increase so that your heart and lungs adapt to your exercise routine. During the rest periods, you don't stop entirely but keep moving at a more gentle pace. When I teach people who are just starting to get back into exercise, this is exactly what I suggest to them.

In my classes, I see many people who have injured themselves with strenuous exercise. Now in their 50s and 60s, they're faced with knee and hip replacements. There are people walking around with their knees scraping bone on bone. Ouch!

Many of us are realizing that the exercise routine that was perfect in our youth may be causing damage later in life. In our younger years we figured that we'd live forever—we pushed our bodies and took huge chances with our health that may not bode well for us now. Distance runners may have great cardiovascular health, for instance, but as they age, they could develop muscle, ligament, and joint problems. Now gyms and fitness centers are starting to cater to the aging physical-fitness enthusiast, featuring equipment and training that focus on balance, strength, and endurance.

I used to do strenuous exercise in my 30s and 40s. I took fitness classes three times a week, and I even did some distance running until I injured my back and spent three months in therapy. Then I slowed down.

I also used to enjoy downhill skiing. There's nothing more exhilarating than sweeping down a freshly groomed hill with a sense of fluidity and freedom. Yet seven years ago, I gave it up, feeling that there was too great a risk of hurting myself—or, more to the point, of some other skier running into me!

For years I've understood that daily exercise is important, but at my age, I'm just not willing to tax my body. To date I have no joint pain, and I can squat down and bend my knees with ease. I consider myself very lucky.

الـه

If you're 50 years of age or older, you may be discovering that your knees are giving out or your muscles ache. It's time to make a switch to fun, effective, and low-impact activities. The body knows how it wants to exercise, and as the years tick by, you'll become more attuned to what its needs are rather than what fitness experts tell you.

Do choose an exercise that you love. For example, in the summer, I swim every day; while in the fall, winter, and spring, I walk. Sometimes I do stretches and yoga poses early in the morning and watch the sun come up.

(**Note:** Please be sure to check with your doctor before embarking on any exercise program. This is especially important if you're over 50, haven't exercised in a

while, have weight problems, or are on medication.)
Here are some fun and safe pursuits:

1. Cross-country skiing. After I quit downhill skiing, I took this up, and it's great exercise that still gives
me that fun, exhilarating feeling, but without the danger. It's also a very social activity: You can climb, ski, and
chat; and then retreat to the log cabin on a crisp winter
evening for hot apple cider. I can enjoy cross-country
skiing for the rest of my life.

2. Swimming. If you like swimming, you can try
jogging in the deep end of the pool. Get yourself a foam
swim belt (it's much like a water-ski belt)—strap that
onto your waist, get into the deep end of the pool, and
start jogging. With this form of exercise, there's no strain
on your back or knees, and you can really work up a
sweat.

I don't use a swim belt anymore, as I just jog and use
my arms to stabilize myself. I swim a few laps and then
jog for 50 revolutions, do a few more laps and 50 jogs.
This breaks up the routine.

Another swimming exercise I like is called "sculling,"
which is a synchronized-swimming movement:

- Float on your back, lift your head up, and
  lift your toes just above the waterline. Focus
  on your toes and move forward in the direction of your toes, not your head. Keep your
  tummy muscles tight.

- Now quickly move your hands counterclockwise in rapid circles, just below the surface

of the water, propelling yourself as if you're rowing a boat. You'll notice that this is a great workout for upper arms and stomach muscles.

3. Pilates, a very popular form of stretching; **ballet;** or **yoga** all help you get in shape without straining yourself. Combined with deep breathing, these are great workouts. (**Note:** Never do any stretching exercise that your body doesn't feel comfortable with. Don't push too far in a stretch—just do what feels right.)

4. Walking. I like to walk early in the morning in my own neighborhood, which gives me a great sense of connection to the wonder of life. All the little sights and sounds are so intriguing, such as a bunny rabbit or even a deer. While I walk, I have gratitude on my lips. I do my best to be in the moment, in full appreciation of the wonders of everything around me, and feeling how blessed I am to be part of it.

Why not try a daily walk for about 15 minutes and feel gratitude in your heart while you do it?

5. Strengthening upper arms. One of the first areas to "go," at least in women, is the upper-arm area. Because we don't use our arms as much as men do, they tend to become flabby and weak. Loose, flaccid muscles in women and men are the result of lack of exercise and hormonal decline.

You never know when you might need to hoist yourself up. Strength in the upper arms could be very valuable, as it is with Vi, my 90-year-old neighbor. She needed to build up her arms to navigate her walker and wheelchair, and she now has amazing upper-arm strength.

If we start exercising our arms now, hopefully we won't need a walker or a wheelchair—but if we do, we'll have the strength to handle it.

Here's a simple upper-arm push-up:

- Stand about four feet away from your bathroom or kitchen counter and place your hands, shoulder-width apart, upon it. Keep your feet flat on the floor, and don't rise up on your toes.

- Use the counter to do some push-ups: Start with 10 if you're huffing and puffing, then increase to 20 after a few days. Keep increasing to 50 per day. You'll notice that you have increased upper-arm strength in about two weeks.

- Add another part to the stretch by "dropping into it": Focus on your upper back by pressing your shoulder blades together during the push-up.

6. Pole walking is another way to get a great workout and build upper-body strength. No, it's not pole *dancing* . . . although that would also be low-impact exercise, and maybe a lot more fun!

Pole walking involves the use of modified ski poles (they don't have the baskets at the ends). As you walk, you extend the pole forward and plant it while your arm is in a handshake position. You then push the pole firmly while stepping forward. You plant the ski poles in opposition to your foot motion—left arm and right leg forward, right arm and left leg forward, and so forth. This motion exercises the upper body, abdominals, and leg muscles.

The poles allow for stability, and even though they're not heavy, there is some resistance due to their weight, thereby exercising wrists as well as arms. (Wearing gloves can help you avoid blisters.) At first you might feel a little self-conscious, but pole walking is really catching on, and I notice more and more people enjoying this form of exercise.

7. Bottoms up! According to my friend Joanie, who just turned 60, "The worst thing about growing older is when you bend down to tie your shoes, you look up and see your butt hanging down between your legs." If this sounds like you, try the "bottoms up" exercise while lying in your bed. It's best done before you go to sleep at night and again before you get out of bed in the morning (I do 50 of these exercises every morning and night). Keeping your back flat, bend your knees and keep your feet flat on the bed. Now tighten your buttocks muscles and tilt your pelvis slightly upward, "pubes" to the sky.

These butt lifts resemble a pelvic tilt, but the buttocks muscles are kept tight. This exercise is great for men and women, as it strengthens the anal-sphincter and bladder muscles, which can loosen with age; strengthens the pelvic floor; helps with urinary incontinence; aids vaginal atrophy; and increases sexual gratification. (Remember that sex is a great workout, too!)

8. DNA movement. You'll love to tone your body with DNA exercise, which is done to music. If you look on the Internet, you can find a selection of musical notes that are correlated to DNA sequences, and these are really quite stunning. The category is called "electronic arts."

On a deeper level, this music is very compelling, rather like the call of dolphins or whales. When you listen to it, you're transported out of your body at a cellular level. You can also choose some nice New Age, spacey music (I love that of artist Hilary Stagg). Look for music with no beat and no particular rhythm.

You'll move your body spontaneously and be completely in tune with every cell—you just let your body stretch and move to the sounds. DNA movement is a terrific workout, one in which you'll feel completely at peace, absorbed by the music, and tuned in to the cells of your body.

Exercise is such a great way to reduce stress. Now let's see how we can improve our digestion, which is another area commonly affected by tension.

CHAPTER 9

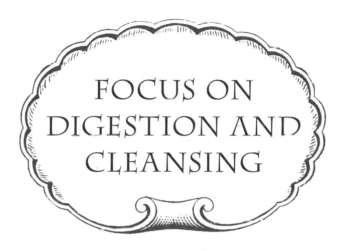

FOCUS ON DIGESTION AND CLEANSING

· ·

As we age, we lose digestive capacity. After the age of 40, hydrochloric-acid production wanes, and we're unable to break down proteins efficiently . . . enter Tums. I remember when my siblings and I were cleaning out our mother's cupboards after she died, and we discovered bottle after bottle of antacids. Some people hoard gold; our mother hoarded Tums.

Most individuals think that the need for antacids is due to the production of too much stomach acid, while the reverse is true. Antacids neutralize one of the body's most important secretions—hydrochloric acid—that, along with the enzyme pepsin, is necessary for protein digestion. Acid blockers make the stomach more alkaline and less acidic than it needs to be; in other words, antacids could actually be blocking the body's ability to digest food, vitamins, and minerals.

Gas and bloating are sure signs of low stomach acid, and there's nothing more socially unacceptable than a good case of "bum gas." If you're living with someone who's constantly got the "toots," I suggest betaine hydrochloride, which is available at health-food stores. This supplement helps neutralize stomach acid, breaks down proteins efficiently, balances PH levels, and stops gas and bloating—a welcome relief to all family members.

You'll also notice a huge difference in your gut when you stop drinking coffee and consuming dairy products, which are probably the main stomach-distress culprits. Over and over again, I find that when people listen to their bodies and put aside offending foods, almost all of their gastrointestinal problems disappear.

Food, Emotions, and Karma

Why is food so important, and why is it pivotal for overall health as we age? I believe it's all about karma.

Karma looks like a wheel, which fans out and encompasses every aspect of your life. If you look at food, it's central to your karmic wheel because in order to live, you must eat. You can look at it like "the house that Jack built": The job that you take to earn the money to buy the food, or the person whom you choose to live with who earns the money to feed you, means that you set karma in motion. The men and women you meet at your job, the contacts you make, and the experiences you have all fan out from this one central aspect of your karmic wheel—food. So let's go into the center of the wheel and do some corrections here.

As the stomach represents power, if you're affected by an emotional issue, you'll feel it there, having a "gut reaction." Over the years, you may have become heavily invested in things that were beyond your control, and you've given away your power or energy to them. Take a look again at your emotional energy tank—is it draining out to an elderly parent, an unsupportive mate, or a financial concern? If you don't have any energy to utilize the nutrients from food, you're going to have stomach problems. After all, if your energy is all drained out, how can you possibly digest food efficiently?

Since digestion breaks down with age, you may also develop multiple food allergies and sensitivities. The way to handle this as you get into your 50s, 60s, and beyond is to eat foods that are more nurturing. "Gut disturbers" such as chili, spicy foods, and acidic items like tomatoes and grapefruit may not be your best bet. And, of course, leave the dairy products alone until you see an improvement.

I have my own food regimen, in which I tune in to my body and give it what it needs. I take digestive enzymes with each meal; I use probiotics or acidophilus to recolonize the flora in my lower colon; I lightly steam my vegetables, even at breakfast; and I never drink juice. I also stay away from tomatoes, since they're too acidic for me at this stage of my life. I like a nice piece of grilled halibut and veggies for dinner, along with some rice or squash. I keep things simple—I use fresh herbs, and I steer clear of complicated sauces where I might encounter hidden food allergies.

If your stomach is delicate, I find that lightly steamed vegetables may be better tolerated than raw. I'm a big fan of soups and stews because they're so nurturing.

You can get an almost instantaneous correction from stomach problems with good old chicken or turkey soup (made without the wheat noodles)—a pot of it on the stove provides a ready source of fuel that will keep everyone happy. Make enough to share with your neighbor or friend who needs some extra TLC.

Cleansing with Water and Oil

Recently a man with stage iv prostate cancer came to me, carrying a large bottle of diet cola. This wasn't nourishing for such a sick man, but he's not alone. Most of us down vats of coffee, soda pop, and alcohol and wonder why we're sick or wrinkled up like prunes.

A big part of your healing journey is going to involve water. There's so much hype regarding this vital liquid: There's spring water, mountain water, artesian water, ionized water, enhanced water, purified water, and special waters from countries all around the world. It's easy to get totally confused about which one is the best to drink.

The other day at my local health-food store, I saw a woman with a case of "enhanced water" in her cart—it had apparently been energized under a pyramid and then charged with negative ions before it was pumped into the bottles. But there she was, strolling along with a double Americano coffee (whew!) in her hand, and I wondered what good this hoopty-doo water was going to do for her. Plus, the bottles were plastic; remember, we now know that plastics can leach dangerous xenoestrogens into our systems and contribute to our toxic estrogen load. This woman would have been much better off with tap water.

I have an under-the-sink filtration system in my kitchen, and when I'm at home I drink eight large glasses of water each day. When I travel I use spring water . . . yes, from plastic bottles. But I consistently detoxify my liver to make sure that unwanted estrogens don't build up in my body.

Sometimes as we age, we don't feel hydrated—we may be drinking enough water, but it doesn't seem to be going into our cells. Perhaps we need to take a look at our electrolytes, ensuring that minerals such as potassium and sodium are in the proper mix. If our digestive systems aren't functioning properly, or if our diet is poor or we live in a hot or humid climate, our electrolyte balance could be compromised.

If you suspect that this is indeed the case, you can purchase an electrolyte solution at a health-food store. When you drink water with added electrolytes, it slakes your thirst, and you can tell that you're better hydrated: Your skin will appear to be more elastic, and the skin on the backs of your hands will snap back instead of staying in peaks when you pinch it.

Please note that symptoms of low blood sugar, hyperinsulinemia, or prediabetes can include constant thirst and a dry mouth—check with your doctor if you're experiencing these symptoms. Adding an electrolyte solution to your water may help, as will balancing blood sugars by eating protein at meals.

Oil Pulling

While we can detoxify the body with water, we can also do it with oil. Have you heard of "oil pulling," which is a technique that originally comes from India? Because I've lived in India, I know that many of the country's mystics and yogis practice some interesting health cures. Not only did yoga itself originate in India, but so did the idea of ingesting a water-soaked cloth to purge the sinuses and digestive tract. The practice of drinking an ounce or two of one's own urine each day to remove toxins is another novel cure that thousands of people in India use on a daily basis. I have a book about it in my library, and it's not going to be everyone's cup of tea (so to speak), but there are evidently numerous health benefits.

The technique of oil pulling is a simple, albeit unusual, healing process in which you swish cold-pressed oil around in your mouth—but don't swallow. The best oils to use are sunflower or sesame, and the procedure should be done before meals and on an empty stomach. It's best to do it before breakfast on a daily basis for a month, and then every second week after that.

Here's the method, which was given to me by Dr. Jim MacKimmie:

1. Take one tablespoon of oil in your mouth, but do not swallow it.

2. Slowly move the oil around in a rinsing, swishing, or pulling motion through the teeth for 15 to 20 minutes. This process thoroughly mixes the oil with your saliva.

3. Apparently, the swishing activates the enzymes that draw toxins out of the blood, and during this pulling process, the oil has become toxic. As the swishing process

continues, the oil becomes thinner and white. If it's still yellow, it hasn't been swished long enough. Again, do not swallow the oil.

4. After the 15 or 20 minutes have passed, spit out the oil. (If you've accidentally swallowed any of it, don't be concerned—it will be expelled through your digestive system.) Thoroughly rinse your mouth with warm tap water.

5. Because what you've spit out contains bacteria and toxins, use antibacterial detergent to clean your sink thoroughly.

The oil-pulling/swishing process is said to improve health and metabolism on all levels. People who have used it have noticed that their gums stop bleeding and their teeth become whiter.

Having a great brain, including sharp memory and optimal mental capacity, is the next topic for our vibrant-aging plan.

CHAPTER 10

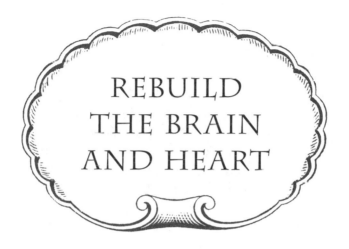

REBUILD THE BRAIN AND HEART

. . . .

Every year I give a medical-intuitive training seminar in which I teach people from all over the world how to tune in to their bodies and improve their health, and I find that they all want to improve their memories. One of the first slides that I put up on the screen in these seminars is of a bottle of "Memory Fix" (not its real name)—it turns out that many in the audience have tried this product, thinking that the way to recover declining memory is to take a few pills. Wrong. I'm very concerned about anyone who buys expensive vitamins in the quest for good health, when simple dietary changes would be more beneficial.

If you want a great memory, you need to work on your gut: Digestive capacity wanes as you grow older, so more toxins enter the body unchecked, and many of them end up in your brain. You also need to take your hormones into account.

Help for the Brain

In my work as a medical intuitive, I've been privileged to meet some of the top researchers and scientists in their fields. One such expert is Dr. Roberta ("Robbie") Diaz Brinton, a neuroscientist, researcher, and professor of molecular pharmacology and toxicology at the University of Southern California in Los Angeles (**http://pharmweb.usc.edu/brinton-lab/**).

After her sister, Eve (whom I mentioned earlier in the book), came to me as a client a few years ago, I had the exciting experience of discussing hormones and memory with Robbie. Her expertise lies in the relationship between Alzheimer's disease and the presence or lack of estrogen. It seems that estrogen is associated with memory, and as we age, its levels decline. Robbie's groundbreaking work explores how estrogen and progesterone could protect against cognitive decline and disease in postmenopausal women, along with increasing the growth of cortical neurons in the brain.

According to Robbie, 68 percent of Alzheimer's patients are women; therefore, if we want to keep our mental faculties, we need to be proactive about balancing our hormones. When I spoke with her, she agreed that diet and nutrition were very important keys to overall brain health. She said that my work was like presenting a "clean canvas" (a detoxified brain) to the body, thus enabling hormone therapy to be more effective, and she was subsequently a presenter at my "Forever Ageless for Men and Women: Anti-Aging Conference."

Since digestive capacity declines over the years, adding digestive enzymes into our daily regimen improves the absorption of nutrition. Nutrients are absorbed through the small intestine and transported through the bloodstream to feed and nourish all parts of the body, including brain cells. If you're looking for a great reference on rebuilding brain cells, take a look at *The Better Brain Book: The Best Tools for Improving Memory and Sharpness and Preventing Aging of the Brain,* by David Perlmutter, M.D., FACN, and Carol Colman (Riverhead).

Dr. Perlmutter is a young renegade neurologist and director of the Perlmutter Health Center in Naples, Florida. He explains that everyday memory lapses such as misplacing car keys, forgetting names, or losing concentration or focus need not be a natural part of aging—in fact, these are actually warning signs of a distressed brain. His recommendations for brain repair include specific supplementation, including B vitamins, N-acetyl-cysteine, acetyl-L-carnitine, lipoic acid, coenzyme Q10, and the herb gingko biloba.

He also recommends removing environmental toxins and chemicals; making dietary and lifestyle changes; and regularly doing brain exercise, such as memory games. Dr. Perlmutter's treatments have been very successful in helping people with memory loss, dementia, and Alzheimer's disease.

One of the important signs of cognitive decline is an inability to make rational decisions, so how's your own brain functioning? Are you becoming forgetful, having difficulty remembering events or people's names?

If you're looking for an improvement in brain function, know that it depends on a number of factors:

- Nutrition—eat healthy food

- Oxygenation—get daily exercise

- Digestion—improve gut flora and enzyme function so that food is digested and utilized

- Supplementation—use products that support brain function

- Elimination—get rid of toxins, which can be carried to the brain through the bloodstream

- Hormone balance—know that studies now show that hormone deficiencies affect memory

- Mental stimulation—stretch brain capacity through books, activities, and the enjoyment of life

All of the above are important for healthy long-term memory.

Memory and Metaphysics

On a higher level, memory loss relates to things or events people don't *want* to remember; in other words, a decline in status or lifestyle or an absence of close friends and loved ones may be too painful to recall. Life can become complicated as time goes by, and some men and women may have a desire to "let go" of their focus and move into that "null zone."

These issues notwithstanding, I believe that having a destiny or purpose—which keeps us young, active, and involved—is a wonderful way to remain youthful. The body knows, and it can respond and bounce back, regardless of our age . . . we just need to give it the tools to do so.

Good memory comes from a healthy diet, supplementation, hormone balancing, oxygenation through exercise, and the desire to learn. An inquisitive mind that's creative and continues to search for knowledge is very important for enhancing memory.

My mother had three college degrees, yet she continued to take courses later in life. She studied Latin and Greek at a university, finally giving up on these challenging studies at age 77—only because she found the heavy classroom doors and the fear of being knocked over by rambunctious students too much for her. But my friend Jane, who just turned 94, is *still* taking courses at the university . . . and she drives to class, too! She gets calls from her "boyfriends" in retirement homes who say, "I'll take you to lunch if you drive." Life is about continuing to learn. As Louise Hay, my mentor and publisher who's now in her 80s, says, "I'm always learning something new."

Rebuilding and Protecting the Heart

Heart health is so important as we age, particularly since more men *and* women in the U.S. die from cardiovascular disease than any other cause. It's estimated that one in four people has some sort of heart-related malady: Hardening of the arteries, heart attacks, irregular heart rhythms, high blood pressure, and strokes account for millions of deaths each year.

The heart is the hearth and life-force center of our bodily home. That's why I'm fascinated by the work of Glenn Alabastro, a specialist in traditional Chinese medicine, who believes that the chi or life force enters through the heart. Alabastro teaches a technique called "heart-rate variability," which involves establishing different breathing patterns, from light and quick to deep and slow. According to Alabastro, testing the breath in relationship to the heart rate can reveal the biological age of a person, which can also be a predictor of heart problems. Testing my own heart-rate variability on similar equipment showed that I have a biological age of 42. Exercising, including climbing stairs, and deep breathing can improve your personal rate. (To learn more, visit: **www.drtranquility.com**.)

Heart issues run in my family: My father died of an aneurism at the age of 61, and my mother passed away at age 87, four years after she had a stroke. I obviously need to be careful with my heart and circulatory system.

My health program started out innocently at the age of 39, and I never knew that healing myself of various imbalances would lead me into a career in complementary medicine and medical intuition. Taking the pressure off of my heart was the first step of my journey. I removed all of the substances that were weakening my body, such as wheat, corn, sugar, coffee, and Baileys Irish Cream. All these things that I loved were making me sick, but once I gave them up, I stopped having heart palpitations, and I slept better. Then I became consistent about eating protein at each meal, and I had red meat at least twice a week, which helped support the electrical firing of my heart.

Next, I limited my sugar intake, knowing that glycation would lay down plaque in my arteries. I learned how to meditate, discovering that serenity was healing, not only for my heart, but for every one of my organs. Then I added in fish oils to my supplement regime—these oils, along with coconut and olive oil, aid in the support of arterial walls. Finally, I discovered oral chelation, which is formulated to break down plaque in the arteries. I started my first oral-chelation program when I was 45, and I've done several of them since.

I love what I do for a living, I take heart-healthy approaches as often as possible, and I do my best to find balance in my life. I'm very grateful for my calming husband, who reminds me not to take things too seriously.

Like me, you may be susceptible to heart problems—and while a poor diet on the physical level is easily remedied, don't neglect the mental level. If you're overtaxed, overburdened, and overworked, you're likely to be disconnected from what you really want to do in life. You're feeding your body negative foods, and feeding your heart negative emotions.

It takes patience and dedication to access the root cause of any issue, including those that have to do with the heart. I'm a big fan of David Rowland, Ph.D., who is a nutritionist and formulator of the oral-chelation product that I use, as well as the author of *The Nutritional Bypass: Reverse Atherosclerosis Without Surgery* (Rowland Publications). Here's what he says about the healing process: "All that healing requires, and the only thing it requires, is to stop the resistance." This is where a personal examination of what's preventing you from experiencing optimal health on all levels of your body, mind, and spirit can come in handy.

Find a quiet corner of your home where you can meditate and feel peaceful. Sit quietly and take a few deep breaths. Relax and open to the inner voice of the Divine within you. With your hand on your heart, make friends with the powerful giant that's beating inside you.

After a few minutes, take out a sheet of paper and a pen and ask yourself what you can do to support your heart. Write down the answers you get to the following:

- Diet—what changes do you need to make?

- Exercise—are you getting enough?

- Stress level—can this be reduced? If so, how?

- Balance—can you create more balance in your life? If so, how?

- Purpose—how can you make life more meaningful?

Healing the Emotional Heart

Now let's look at the emotional heart, which is where the deepest level of personal self-mastery resides.

There are a lot of emotional heart-related issues that run in my family as well, and I wasn't able to scale my own mountain until I could deal with them. Maybe you're like me, and you perceive that you had a difficult childhood. Perhaps you weren't heard as a child, weren't validated, or didn't feel loved and appreciated. If that sounds like you, I hope you'll be able to relate to my story of forgiveness.

For as long as I could remember, my mother and I hadn't been close. Of course she loved me, and I'm sure that she held me when I was little, but growing up and on into adulthood, I never felt connected to her. I always envied my girlfriends' relationships with their mothers. I'd look at the spark between two generations of women—the sharing, laughing, and confiding—and wish I had that. My mom and I seemed to try to meet, but it never really happened.

As time wore on, I abandoned any idea of a meaningful relationship with her. Happily, I married and gave birth to two beautiful daughters with whom I'm very close. Now adults themselves, I consider them my best friends. This, I reasoned, was worth the distance that I felt with my own mother. *Still,* I thought, *wouldn't it be wonderful if there could be a healing between Mom and me before she died?*

Every night for 15 years, I sent a loving prayer to my mother, which was the least I could do. I tried to focus on the positive things I felt about her, such as her courage since the death of my father; her independence and desire to do things for herself; her love of classical music; and, most important, her strong faith and regular church attendance, which made up the foundation of my own spirituality.

One day, before I was to leave for a speaking engagement, I got a panicked call from my sister: "Come quick! Mom's in the emergency ward—she's just had a stroke." As I sped to the hospital, I thought, *Okay, this is it. Maybe she'll just die, and this whole thing will be over.* When I got there, I peered over the steel bars on her bed and saw this pale, frail woman, who was seemingly comatose. I said a silent prayer, *Thy will be done, O Lord.*

"She's had a massive stroke," the doctor told me, "and her whole left side has been affected. Fortunately, we have her on a brand-new IV procedure designed to break up the clot in her carotid artery, which is affecting the flow of oxygen to her brain. Let's hope it works."

I looked down at Mom, whose eyes were fluttering, and wondered if she'd ever speak to us again.

"Squeeze my hand, Mary," the nurse said to my mother. No response. "Lift your leg," she encouraged. No response. We all waited, watched, and chatted with low voices and grave faces, while the IV monitor blipped its vital signs. The nurse tried again. "Mary," she asked, "who is that standing beside you?"

"That's my daughter Caroline," she said in a clear voice.

"Can you squeeze my hand with your left one?" Mom did so perfectly. "Lift your left leg." No problem. It was a miracle: Just 20 minutes before, things had looked bleak—now my mother was responding well.

Shortly after this near-fatal stroke, my mom was living in her own home and gaining strength. She used a walker and was wobbly and frail, but she was determined. And a whole new chapter was written for us. Gone was the brittle, distant woman with her judgments and criticism. Gone was the person I resented visiting. I welcomed my mother into my heart.

Miraculously, *The Evolution Angel: An Emergency Physician's Lessons with Death and the Divine* by Dr. Michael Abrams (Abundance Media) came into my hands during this time. A concept in the book that stood out for me was that each person begs—yes, begs—to be born.

This idea that I'd begged to be born of this woman transported me to a deeper level of healing, along with an appreciation of my mother.

The metaphysics of this relationship were obviously very karmic. The goal of the universe is that our birth families provide the ideal backdrop for the evolution of our souls. So my mother and father were the perfect parents for me—throughout my younger life, the lack of connection with them was deeply wounding, but it led me to establish deep bonds with many other people and to be a healing presence for them.

After I read that section in Dr. Abrams's book, I decided to go and spend time with my mother a little differently. I visited her after dinner, and I carefully brushed her dentures, washed her face, and got her ready for bed. I made this into a spiritual practice, recognizing her for her role and for giving me life. Then we did Vespers together. I took out her Bible, hymnal, and prayer book; we looked up the psalm of the day, and my mother read it. Then we read Bible passages, and we marked favorite hymns and sang them together. It was an incredibly bonding time, and I let my intuition lead me.

Mom and I didn't know how much time she had left on the planet, but we had a wonderful time together. I could stroke her hair, kiss her cheek, hold her hand, and tell her I loved her—and I meant it. Our relationship was an answer to a prayer. It was a pleasure to be with her and even run her errands.

Once when I took her swimming, the lifeguard lowered the handicapped chair into the pool. As I helped my mother out of the chair and into the water, I held her in my arms. I looked up and said "Thank You, God. At last I have a mother."

My mom lived for another four years, and we spent many happy days together. It took all that time for me to love and forgive her for her human failings, along with her lack of support or acknowledgment of my intuitive gifts. As she was progressing on her spiritual journey, I was progressing on mine.

When she died, two weeks before her 88th birthday, my sister and I were by her side. The healing job was done—Mom and I were both at peace.

In reviewing this situation with the knowledge I currently possess, I know that a large part of my mother's personality peculiarities were hormonally related. She was a healthy, vital woman who had a child relatively late in life. I recall an incident while she and my father were living in India when she was rushed to the hospital late one night with excessive bleeding—I realize now that she suffered from a progesterone deficiency, which can be a reason for heavy bleeding. When a woman is estrogen dominant and progesterone deficient, she can become anxious, bitchy, mean, and nasty. Through no fault of her own—and a tragic medical oversight—my mother's symptoms were never treated.

I hope that my story will help you ponder your own life and relationships more deeply.

Next, let's focus on ways to get you healthy, renew your vitality and stamina, and keep you out of the cancer zone.

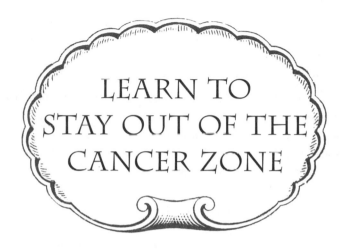

CHAPTER 11

LEARN TO STAY OUT OF THE CANCER ZONE

• •

You've probably noticed that young people don't get cancer in the same numbers that older people do. Cancer is indeed a predominantly age-related illness—the lifestyle of an aging person could be placing him or her at risk for the disease.

As a medical intuitive, I'm shocked by how many people are walking around with precancerous conditions. One in five individuals are predicted to develop cancer, which is a very scary statistic. Not that long ago the average life span was 57 years; now it's 79. Since we're living longer, if we're not careful, there are more years in which we can develop diseases.

This chapter will reveal insights and strategies to help keep you out of the cancer zone. Let's begin with a tale from a very inspirational lady.

Jodie's Story

I saw Jodie across a crowded meeting room several years ago at Marianne Williamson's church in Detroit, and I had to speak to her. Something compelled me to tell the people who were in line to meet me to wait—I needed to talk to someone. Like a compass, my intuition guided me to a pale, frail woman seated at the back of the room. I sat on the arm of her chair, held her hand, and listened to her story. This is what happened, in Jodie's own words:

> I was in the middle of chemotherapy, along with 35 heavy-duty radiation treatments on my chest wall and 11 more on my right hip, and I was very weak and using a wheelchair. A pediatric cardiologist friend of mine called and asked if there was any way I could attend a seminar given by Caroline Sutherland, which could change the course of my illness toward recovery. It seems that Caroline was coming to my church the following weekend— the universe couldn't have orchestrated this meeting more perfectly. I agreed to go.
>
> My friend told me to sit in the back of the room; not to make eye contact; and, for heaven's sake, not to ask Caroline a question or she might bring me up to the front of the room.
>
> It wouldn't have mattered where I sat or what I did, for this diminutive, energetic woman was drawn to me like a magnet. Across a room of several hundred people, she found me, and as she sat on the arm of my chair, I heard words that would orient my healing compass in a completely different direction.
>
> I told Caroline that I was 59 years old, and my life had been a series of twists and turns. Two years after undergoing a divorce (after 35 years of marriage), I was

diagnosed with stage iv breast cancer and metastatic bone disease. I'd lost 28 people to cancer in my close family, so I had many difficult decisions to make.

I chose all the best doctors and researched everything that I could pertaining to my illness. Chemotherapy and radiation—and all of the side effects that come with them—became part of my daily life. Forty-six pounds had fallen off my body at this point, and I'd begun to seriously explore complementary medicine . . . and that's when I met Caroline.

I attended all of her workshops that weekend in Detroit, and I felt the first glimmer of hope that I could regain my strength and energy. As Caroline sat with me and shared what she felt was out of balance, she outlined a plan of action with dietary recommendations, supplementation, Candida-yeast control, and food-allergy elimination. I embarked upon the program right away and began to feel much stronger. Her beef-broth recipe [found on page 288] seemed to be a magical elixir, and I drank the South American medicinal tea that she recommended. I started to feel a strength that amazed my doctor and me.

I added vitamins, herbs, and an immune-enhancing blender drink—I was finally able to eat more than applesauce and water, which for weeks had been all I could keep down. I then found an environmental nutritionist who immediately started me on intravenous vitamin C to stimulate my immune system and strengthen my body.

Since I had numbness and no range of motion in my right arm as a result of the radiation treatments, acupuncture was the next part of my protocol. After a month of weekly treatments, my right arm was so improved that my doctors were simply astounded.

Then I decided to attend the Women's Midlife Journey Program at the beautiful Canyon Ranch spa in Lenox, Massachusetts. I began with two superb instructors who gave me back the gift of exercise with the yoga and Pilates that I'd always loved.

I also chose to participate in some "healing touch" sessions during that week at Canyon Ranch, which totally shifted my perceptions about my divorce and illness. Imagine healing from the heartbreak of loving a man whom I'd first met when I was 14 years old. It was as if he'd died, and I was now coming out of a deep state of post-traumatic stress disorder—the aftermath of my own personal 9/11. During this time I read Catherine Ponder's book *The Dynamic Laws of Healing* (DeVorss), which deals with forgiveness and healing practices, and I did a lot of journaling. All of this really helped.

Today, I'm in what's called "remission," but I am 100 percent cancer free. By combining the best of traditional and complementary medicine, I've become a walking miracle.

Not long ago, I took a Rolex watch that my ex-husband had given me into the jeweler. It had always been my favorite, but I wanted to have the bezel changed. I asked to have diamonds put into it, one for each of the tests that I'd undergone these past four years: courage, patience, healing, understanding, love, forgiveness, and so forth. Then I asked to have four sapphires set—one each at 12, 3, 6, and 9—representing dignity, integrity, health, and happiness. Every day this new watch face reminds me of how far I've come. I can now walk on the beach, feel the breeze on my face, and breathe in the sea air; and I appreciate each day that I live with joy and gratitude.

By tuning in to Jodie when I met her, I knew that her will or desire to keep going was teetering in the balance. There's a fine line between life and death, and I didn't feel that there was much time to capture the thread of wellness that still remained within her body and pull her back into life.

Often a cancer diagnosis can be preceded by a cataclysmic event. In Jodie's case, her immune system had taken a strong hit when the shock of finding her husband of 35 years with a younger woman rocked her emotional foundation. She was laid to waste emotionally, and was unprotected physically . . . so it wasn't surprising that her body had developed a life-threatening illness.

When a person is weak, he or she needs nurturing, and soup often comes to me as a remedy for such an individual. So as I held Jodie's hand, I tuned in to her and said, "You are severely depleted. I sense that you need beef broth, and plenty of it, along with some very special tea." I'm so glad she listened to me, as well as to her own intuition, and gave her body and soul the chance to completely heal.

Jodie's in remission now, and I was happy to visit her recently in her beautiful vacation home on the beach in California. Her purpose is to enjoy each day of her life, to spread love wherever she goes, and to inspire others with her message that cancer can be overcome.

Some Surprising Facts about Cancer

Before we go any further, I'd like you to think about the following salient points, which have come from a well-known medical school (but have been adapted and modified):

1. From time to time, every person has cancer cells in his or her body, but they may not appear in standard

medical tests. Following treatment, when a patient is told that he or she is in remission, this term applies to *detectable* cancer. In other words, undetected cancer cells could still exist in the body.

2. Cancer cells appear several times during a person's life. Usually these abnormal cells are engulfed by the immune system and destroyed through the process of *apoptosis,* or natural cell death. This prevents cancer cells from multiplying or forming tumors.

3. Cancer is a multifaceted disease. So nutritional deficiencies, food intolerance, yeast overgrowth, environmental issues, stress, hormonal imbalances, and genetic and lifestyle factors can all influence the growth of cancerous cells.

4. Cancer cells are glucose supported, so an effective defense against their proliferation is to starve them by decreasing sugars in all forms (and avoiding the consumption of milk products, which are mucus forming).

5. Cancer cells can become resistant to treatment or, as the result of surgery, spread to other parts of the body.

6. Cancer treatment should include stress reduction, dietary changes, lifestyle modifications, and specific immune-building supplementation; that is, both traditional and nontraditional approaches.

7. The favored traditional cancer treatment is chemotherapy, which is designed to destroy fast-growing

cancer cells, but it can also affect healthy cells and may cause damage to organs and systems.

8. Toxic load from either chemotherapy or radiation affects the immune system and may expose the cancer patient to complications or infections.

9. Initial cancer treatment with chemotherapy and radiation may often reduce tumor size. However, prolonged use of these treatments may result in tumor recurrence in other areas of the body, or cancer cells could proliferate due to toxicity or the body's weakened defense mechanisms.

10. Radiation is designed to destroy cancer cells, but it can also burn, scar, and damage healthy cells, tissues, and organs. Hyperbaric treatment, which increases the transportation of oxygen in the blood and improves the activity of white blood cells, can be useful for healing after the effects of chemotherapy and radiation.

11. Finally, I'd like to introduce you to an innovative form of cancer treatment called "insulin potentiation therapy" (IPT) that bears investigating. Patients are given low-dose chemotherapy that has minimal side effects, along with insulin to balance erratic blood-sugar levels. Several of my clients have undergone IPT, with very favorable results—they said that they immediately felt better and had more energy, thanks to the stabilized blood sugar. As an important strategy to stay out of the cancer zone, IPT patients are not only encouraged to stay away from sugar, but to also do their all-important forgiveness work. (Please visit: **www.iptq.org**.)

Sugar and Cell Death

Reproduction and death are built into every living thing's system. The salmon returns to the same river each year to lay her eggs and then die. The mother goat has a baby, and after a few more reproductive cycles, she dies, too. Even trees release seed pods, which flourish elsewhere, and after a time those trees fall over and die.

When we slow down the aging process, we arrest the body's genetic program to reproduce and die, and our focus then becomes repair and regeneration to control our cell destiny. The cell actually has four destinies: (1) to remain alive without dividing, (2) to grow and divide, (3) to regenerate and repair, or (4) to die. Optimal health is achieved when a balance between cell proliferation and cell death is maintained. You see, our body is composed of more than 100 trillion cells, and throughout our life span, those cells that are no longer healthy or useful are engulfed by the immune system. Cancers form when there's uncontrolled cell proliferation and no natural cell death (or apoptosis).

As I mentioned, cancer is a multifaceted disease. Stress, a weakened immune system, hormone imbalances, a toxic environment, or a victim consciousness or deeply held resentment can each contribute to a predisposition to cancer, but sugar is a very important piece of the puzzle.

Did you know that there are currently about 700 medications in use for cancer treatments? Not 7, not 70, but approximately *700*—there are more than 400 in circulation, and more than 200 in the research stages. Wouldn't you think that someone would tell the general public that if they minimized their sugar (and starch) consumption, their cancer risk would go down? It baffles me that this information is not mainstream.

My husband is an oncology nurse. Every day he cares for people with cancer and administers drugs to them. He subscribes to several professional oncology-nursing publications, all of which are sponsored by drug companies. Every month I scour those journals, looking for a thread of truth among all the drug-related jargon. Only once did I see an article entitled "Could Cancer and Obesity Be Related?" Yet it held no major revelations and, of course, the end of it contained the classic line "this subject warrants further study." It seems obvious to me that our society's high obesity rate and cancer statistics are related.

Another method of confirming that cancer cells are glucose supported is the positron-emission tomography (PET) scan, which is an imaging device used in nuclear medicine. The scan produces a three-dimensional map of functional processes in the body and is an accurate way of detecting cancer cells or assessing cancer growth in the body.

The process involves the injection of radioactive isotopes and glucose into the body, and the unique scanning device then takes images of the patient from head to toe. Radioactive chemicals emit wavelengths that can be measured, so the images are carefully observed to see just where the glucose and radioactive isotopes will travel.

Glucose is first observed in the brain, which is to be expected—it's the fuel that allows the brain to think and send messages to the parts of the body where functions are to be performed. Next, glucose is observed in the liver, where it's stored in the form of glycogen, which the body will draw on for its energy supply.

What happens next is what really interests the oncologist or cancer specialist. As the PET scans the rest of the body, it's observed that the glucose and radioactive isotopes go directly and attach themselves to existing cancer cells. This is how new cancers are located or how a patient can be determined to be cancer free. The oncologist's explanation for this is that fast-growing cells need sugar for survival; that is, cancer cells are glucose supported. Stay out of the cancer zone—stop consuming sugar!

Keys for Staying Cancer Free

Take a look at your diet: Is it heavy on sugars and carbs? Carbohydrates convert into sugar in the body, which means that the pizza, pasta, rice, and bread you love so much—in addition to the cookies, cake, candy, and ice cream—convert into glucose. Remember, glucose goes directly to cancer cells. Even juices, honey, and fruit (be it dried or fresh) are all sugar; and a vegetarian diet, unless it's well managed with adequate protein, contains too much starch and sugar.

I remember sitting on a plane next to a cancer survivor once. She was overweight, and as she snacked on bananas and orange juice during the four-hour flight, I couldn't help but feel appalled. This was *not* proactive nutrition, which would help keep her free of a possible recurrence of the disease.

Again, it's worth mentioning Candida albicans, a strain of yeast that's found in the digestive tract and other moist mucous membranes of the body. Candida is one of the great plagues of our culture, and it thrives on starch and sugar. People who suffer from an overgrowth of this yeast experience fatigue, a craving for sweets and carbohydrates, and a host of other symptoms. And major diseases such as lupus, cancer, AIDS, Alzheimer's, chronic fatigue disease, and multiple sclerosis often have Candida in their symptom profile.

Here are some practical strategies to keep yeasts— and cancer—at bay:

- Eradicate the "bad guy" yeasts with natural remedies such as pau d'arco, grapefruit-seed extract, caprylic acid, oregano oil, or garlic.

- Supplement with "good guy" Lactobacillus acidophilus cultures to strengthen the healthy bacteria in the intestines.

- Keep sugars low, having no more than one sweet dessert per week.

- Keep protein consistent, as it starves the little rascals. If protein is eaten at every meal and snack, then blood sugar will also be balanced.

- Limit alcohol to no more than two or three ounces per week.

- Minimize fruit to one piece per day.

- Consume lots of fresh vegetables, especially the colorful, antioxidant-loaded ones.

- Use immune-building supplements.

- Do your forgiveness work—don't hang on to old stuff.

- Love life and *yourself.*

Using Life's Sweetness to Keep Young and Healthy

According to my medical textbook *Principles of Anatomy & Physiology,* by Gerard J. Tortora and Sandra R. Grabowski (Wiley), "Glucose, the most abundant sugar in the body, plays a role in the aging process. As it is added to proteins inside and outside of cells, glucose forms irreversible cross connections, which contribute to stiffening and loss of elasticity in aging skin. Glucose and free radicals damage and contribute to wrinkled skin, stiff joints, and hardened arteries."

This important subject had already made perfect sense to me, and to see it described in a medical textbook brought it into even sharper focus. Sugar and subsequent cell breakdown had come to me intuitively, and I have to thank Dr. Ron Rosedale (whom I discussed earlier in the book) for confirming what I already sensed. He knew the real secret to fighting the war on cancer.

Unfortunately, despite all the fund-raisers, the walk-athons, and the pink lapel ribbons, there are more people diagnosed with cancer today than ever before. Might our starch- and sugar-laden diets have something to do with these statistics?

The big pharmaceutical companies don't want to cure cancer—there are just too many dollars at stake for them. In my opinion, the war on cancer won't be won with some miracle drug or millions of research dollars, but with a few simple strategies and revealing truths.

This was confirmed for me when I met Alma, a top biomedical researcher for a large pharmaceutical company. After our consultation, I asked her about sugar and cancer growth. "Oh yes," she replied, "it's well known that any fast-growing cell needs glucose or sugar to live. This is common knowledge to any scientist."

Then I inquired as to why the public wasn't made aware of this fact, and she responded, "While it isn't news to the scientific community, it's just not spoken of in public circles."

As you can see, in order to prevent the diseases of aging, you need to evaluate your consumption of sugar and refined starches, and encourage apoptosis. Sugar contributes to cell reproduction and prevents cell regeneration and repair. And cancer cells are glucose supported. Isn't it interesting that the very substance you crave and find satisfying is actually causing your body to break down? It's all tied together.

It's ironic that sweet foods represent what's missing in our lives: fulfillment in our work, spiritual vocation, and personal relationships. When we consume sugar to excess, it's actually replacing life's sweetness, thus accelerating the subconscious death wish.

What's the solution? We must build up the immune system with positive thoughts and actions, and obviously reduce the sugars and excessive carbohydrates that feed yeasts and cause cell proliferation and breakdown. Finally, we need to balance hormones, which help protect our bodies from disease, rebuild cells, and replenish our skin.

In the next section of the book, you're going to become familiar with the fascinating world of hormones.

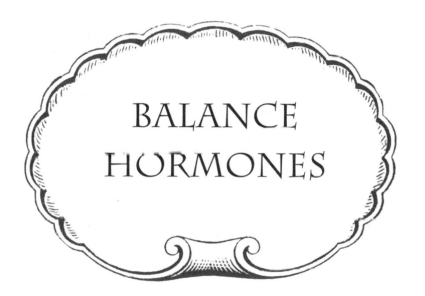

PART III

BALANCE
HORMONES

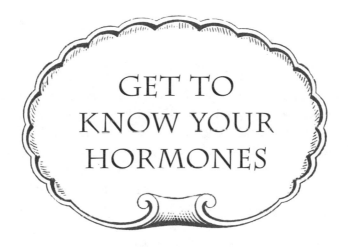

CHAPTER 12

GET TO
KNOW YOUR
HORMONES

• •

Hormones are chemical messengers that course through the bloodstream, interfacing between cells to deliver information. The functions of each gland—from the thyroid and parathyroid to the pituitary, hypothalamus, and pineal glands—and reproductive organ are mediated by this hormone delivery of information. As a matter of fact, our entire body is dependent on proper hormone function and would die within minutes without them.

In this chapter, you're going to become acquainted with your hormones, as well as understand the role they play in a vibrant-aging plan.

Key Hormones

Let's get to know the most important messengers of the human body:

1. Estrogen (which consists of estradiol, estrone, and estriol) is produced in the ovaries, fat cells, and adrenal glands. This hormone is involved in all phases of the growth and regeneration of the female endocrine system: It regulates a woman's reproductive life, including her periods and pregnancies, on through the various stages of menopause. A woman's curves are related to estrogen production, as this is involved in the development of breasts and body fat (as well as body hair). Estrogen also supports healthy tissue in the uterus and urinary tract, and it's even the major hormone associated with memory function. If we women have too little of it, we start to lose our memory.

2. Progesterone is produced in women's ovaries and adrenal glands (and in men's testes), and it protects nerve and brain cells and promotes relaxation and sleep. Progesterone stimulates new bone formation; regulates a woman's menstrual cycle; and prevents miscarriages, thus keeping a pregnancy viable.

3. Testosterone is produced in a woman's ovaries and a man's testes. It helps with endurance; builds lean body mass; protects against arterial plaque; and improves libido, balance, and coordination. It also promotes long-term feelings of security, positivity, and well-being.

4. Thyroid hormone is produced in the thyroid gland and is involved in body temperature, fat-burning metabolism, mood regulation, digestive function, and hair growth.

5. Dehydroepiandrosterone (DHEA) is produced in the adrenal glands and is a building block for cell regeneration, sex-hormone function, and cortisol-level balancing. There are DHEA supplements that can be purchased over the counter; however, do not take them unless you've been tested and found to be deficient in this hormone.

6. Insulin, a growth hormone produced in the pancreas, is responsible for blood-sugar handling. Just by reducing carbohydrates in the diet, you can balance your insulin levels—and when they're normalized, energy goes up.

7. Human growth hormone (HGH) is produced in the pituitary gland. Adequate levels build muscle tone; improve bone density and skin elasticity; increase stamina, energy, and mental clarity; and bring about an optimistic attitude. For some people, HGH is a vital part of a healthy-aging program.

8. Adrenaline is produced by the adrenal glands and protects the body from the effects of stress. This is the hormone secreted during our fight-or-flight reactions.

9. Cortisol is also produced in the adrenal glands, and it's involved in the regulation of sugar (carbohydrate) metabolism. Stress reactions can suppress the immune system, as can too much sugar, making a person more susceptible to infection.

10. Melatonin is produced in the pineal gland and is involved in sleep regulation. If there's too little melatonin in your body, you may wake up in the wee hours of the morning. Supplementation of this hormone may be useful to reestablish sleep patterns after international travel.

All of these hormones work together in concert, so when one is "off," it will affect all the rest. Balancing is key.

The Thyroid and Other Glands

Let's shift our attention to glands for a moment. The hypothalamus is an important endocrine gland that governs appetite, emotion, memory, and hormone balance. The pineal gland responds to light and holds the "master clock," so when darkness falls, we tend to get sleepy. The pituitary gland relates to growth; helps us turn food into energy, therefore having some control over our weight; and regulates blood pressure, appetite, and breast-milk production. The thyroid gland, which is located at the base of the neck, regulates mood, temperature, weight control, and waste elimination.

Many people suffer from glandular trouble, including what's known as "subclinical low thyroid." This is when the level of the thyroid hormone appears just above the bottom of the test range, but it's still seen as normal. Yet even though health-care professionals may not consider the level low enough to require treatment, a person with subclinical low thyroid can feel sluggish and tired.

As a medical intuitive, I see low thyroid as a soft gray haze with an oily quality to it in the aura or electromagnetic field. As soon as I see this oily energetic cast around a person, I know that he or she may be having mood, temperature, or fat-burning issues.

Doctors call the condition of low thyroid "hypothyroidism," and it has reached epidemic proportions in the United States. Since a medical test may not always detect low thyroid, if you suspect that yours is indeed low, purchase a basal thermometer. Take your temperature before you get out of bed each morning for a week, and record your findings. If it's consistently low, in the 96- or 97-degree range (it should be around 98.6), let your practitioner know.

Your naturopathic or holistic physician will be able to determine supplementation based on your symptoms and your temperature chart. Then by using certain herbs, botanicals, glandular materials, or synthetic medication, this important gland will be helped to produce the thyroid hormone again.

For many people, it's as if the lights go on, and the body's energy and fat-burning capacity go up, after the thyroid is balanced. This brings to mind Ruth, a 52-year-old woman I consulted with not long ago. I took one look at her photograph and just knew that her thyroid was low. She'd suspected it herself, but when her doctor tested her, she fell into the "normal" range (albeit near the bottom end). This woman was 50 pounds overweight, and if her thyroid condition continued to be left unchecked, her fat-burning metabolism would continue to suffer.

Now let's look at the metaphysics of what the thyroid represents. It's located at the base of the neck, at the "expression level" or throat area, which corresponds to the ability to speak your truth. Take a look at what you'd like to express, whether it be through your own creativity or by speaking to a person in your life—are you holding back from communicating something that you really need to?

In Ruth's case, she was very unhappy because her 15-year-old son was the only thing keeping her marriage together, and she had difficulty sharing her pent-up frustrations. While on the outside she appeared to be outgoing and in control, she felt alone and sad on the inside. She dulled the pain of her unexpressed feelings with food, and thanks to that and her underactive thyroid, she gained quite a bit of weight. Happily, she was able to take most of it off after she confronted her feelings and balanced her thyroid.

Understanding Cholesterol

As we age, cholesterol becomes a major factor in our pursuit of optimal health. As pointed out by Steve Ayre, a wonderful doctor who practices integrative medicine outside of Chicago (he also utilizes IPT, which I discussed in the last chapter), cholesterol isn't "officially" a hormone because it doesn't perform any particular messenger roles. However, it is the substance in our bodies from which we make pregnenolone, which is part of our sex hormones. (Please visit: **www.contemporarymedicine.net**.)

It's important to understand that cholesterol is formed in our bodies from carbohydrate chains, not fat. The cholesterol that we eat from animal fat is metabolized by the body, and we don't absorb any other. What our doctors measure is the cholesterol we've manufactured, regardless of fat intake. In other words, if we eat a high-cholesterol food, that cholesterol won't become part of our system.

We really need to be more concerned with insulin. This hormone is produced in a part of the pancreas called the islets of Langerhans, and it regulates carbohydrate (starch and sugar) metabolism. Insulin also affects fat metabolism, as it changes the liver's activity from storing to releasing glucose (sugar) as needed for energy and in processing blood lipids. The amount of insulin in circulation has widespread effects throughout the whole body. Since it is considered to be a growth hormone, lowering its levels through the reduction of carbohydrates will contribute to improved hormone function

Cholesterol is a vitally important component in the hormone-balance equation. With the very best of intentions, many people greatly reduce fats in the diet and often affect critical hormone function in the process. And many men and women take statins, which are prescription drugs used to lower cholesterol levels in those who have heart problems or are at risk for cardiovascular disease. Cholesterol-lowering medications are big business in our society: The most popular statin sells more than $12 billion worth of the drug worldwide, and it's among the most commonly prescribed medication in the U.S. today.

Statins lower cholesterol by inhibiting an enzyme that is related to the way cholesterol is formed. Results from using statin drugs can be seen after one week of use, and the effect is maximal after four to six weeks . . . that is, if you want to take them that long. Side effects include gastrointestinal problems, muscle degeneration, joint pain, memory impairment, depression, and kidney or liver failure.

According to my research, reducing cholesterol may not be necessary—it may even be harmful, since fats from animal and vegetable sources form necessary building blocks for cell membranes and a variety of hormone processes. There's also a new theory that high cholesterol is *not* the cause of heart attacks and that saturated fat is healthy—and when I needed confirmation of this theory, the universe sent it right to me.

In *The Doctor's Heart Cure* (Dragon Door Publications), cardiologist Al Sears clearly states that we should dump our high-starch, low-fat eating plans; and that our Paleolithic (hunter/gatherer) ancestry predisposes us to be meat and fat eaters. He cites the Eskimos and the French as having much lower rates of heart disease, even though they have fat-laden diets. According to Sears, obesity rates in the United States began to climb right after all those health experts told us to switch to a low-fat diet.

This information flies in the face of another interesting book. *The China Study,* by T. Colin Campbell, Ph.D., and Thomas Campbell (Benbella Books), shows startling evidence that a vegetable-protein diet can be protective against heart attacks and cancer. But this study was conducted in China, where people have consumed soy and beans as a regular part of their diet for millions of years.

Since its release, *The China Study* has been criticized because of possibly biased statistical conclusions. While people often reference this book as a positive source of information, much of the material may be politically motivated, as Campbell was pro-vegetarian before he did this work. And although he suggests that those he researched ate soybeans for centuries, he fails to point out that they usually consumed *fermented* soy products. This is an important distinction, since plain, raw soy can cause digestive upsets and metabolic imbalances if used over time.

While I'm not a big fan of a strict vegetarian diet, the ethical issues around animal slaughtering are valid. Do your best to purchase organic, hormone-free meats and poultry; and look for farms that institute humane animal-husbandry practices.

There are millions of healthy vegetarians in the world. But I intuitively sense that the proteins they consume often lack essential amino acids; moreover, in time, such a diet can make them weak and tired. Indeed, the most common problem that I used to see in my clinical days, and still do in my readings now, is depleted vegetarians. Therefore, I find that by expanding protein choices (perhaps by adding some fish into the diet), energy and stamina return. Remember that protein is the building block of the cell, so it's a necessary part of any eating plan.

Recent reports indicate that pure vegetarians don't necessarily live longer than anyone else does . . . after all, humans *are* omnivores. Herbivores or plant-eating animals have substances in their bodies that help them convert plant materials into the protein they need, but humans lack those substances. And a vegetarian diet would probably kill a carnivore—a lion, tiger, or bear just wouldn't make it on a vegetables-only regimen. I remember putting our cat on a diet of rice and vegetables once, and he lost all his hair and got very sick. Once meat was added back into the diet, however, he returned to normal and had a beautiful, silky coat.

One thing I will say in favor of T. Colin Campbell's thesis is that he's concerned about dairy product consumption and the link to cancer. Over and over again throughout my career as a medical intuitive, I've seen people who are intolerant of products made from cow's milk, resulting in myriad health problems.

Fat Is Your Friend!

Cholesterol forms vital *corticosteroids,* which are hormones that help us deal with stress and protect our bodies against heart disease and cancer. Cholesterol is also a precursor to the sex hormones androgen, testosterone, estrogen, and progesterone. Put another way, fat can make you feel sexy. Look at the French, with their diets that are loaded with fat—they certainly don't seem to be lacking in the romance department!

Fats in the diet provide energy, along with that sated, not-hungry feeling. In addition, fats act as carriers for several fat-soluble vitamins, including A, D, E, and K; and the assumption that we should reduce their intake could lead to a number of metabolic imbalances. If I'm hungry between meals, I take a tablespoon of coconut oil—a healthy, highly saturated (that is, hard at room temperature) fat. My hunger is satisfied, and my blood sugar is immediately balanced.

I love the work of biochemist and nutritionist Dr. Mary Enig, the author (along with Sally Fallon) of *Eat*

Fat, Lose Fat (Penguin), and she can set us straight on fats. She's been working in "the fat forefront" for more than 25 years, and her protests against trans fats are finally being heard. Mary and Sally confirm in their book what I already knew: that saturated or animal fats constitute at least 50 percent of the cells' membranes. These fats give our cells the necessary strength and integrity to be able to assimilate sugars, as well as to absorb calcium into our skeletal structure.

Healthy fats are the ones you love to eat, including butter; olive, coconut, palm, and flaxseed oil; avocados; and nuts and seeds. And if you can believe it, chicken, duck, and goose fat (which is loved and used by the French) are all very healthy, according to Mary Enig.

Keep in mind that when we were growing up, most of our fat sources came from butter, lard, tallow, coconut oil, and small amounts of olive oil; and there was much less heart disease back then. In the early 1950s, the big deal was margarine—I even remember my mother blending a little yellow disk of coloring into a pound of margarine to make it look like butter. This new spread was subsequently touted as being able to lower cholesterol and prevent heart attacks . . . which couldn't be further from the truth.

Today most of the fats in our diet are derived from vegetable oils (soy, corn, safflower, and canola), and it's almost impossible to find any products at the grocery store that don't contain them. I spent a great deal of time one day searching for a good salad dressing—one after the other was made with soy oil. It was practically inescapable! I now only use olive oil, a little balsamic vinegar, and a sprinkling of fresh herbs in a dressing that I make myself.

These popular fats are very unhealthy. You see, so-called light oils affect the cell walls' ability to process glucose, so the cells' ability to assimilate sugar and starch is lessened. It's bad enough that we have too much starch and sugar in our diets, but if our cell walls are weakened by the wrong kinds of fat, we aren't able to assimilate the starch and sugar at all.

Diabetes and hyperinsulinemia (problems handling sugar in the blood) have now reached epidemic proportions . . . sadly, even among children. I have to scratch my head when I look in people's grocery carts and see packages of cookies and muffins with big signs reading No CHOLESTEROL! It isn't the fat that's making people fat—it's the *wrong kind* of fat, not to mention the amount of starch and sugar in packaged items.

Next, let's apply our knowledge of hormones and learn how to detect an imbalance.

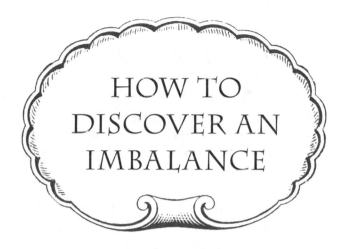

CHAPTER 13

HOW TO DISCOVER AN IMBALANCE

People often ask me how I got involved in bioidentical or natural hormone balancing. I like to reply that I'm always ready for the universe to deliver the next step in my healing journey. Perhaps my story will inspire you to find a balance within your own system.

Hormones and Me

When I'd just turned 60, I went to my doctor's office for a routine checkup. I mentioned that I wasn't feeling quite myself: I'd noticed that my memory wasn't quite as sharp, I was feeling a little bitchy, and I'd been having trouble losing weight. He told me that it might be the right time to take a look at hormone balancing, suggesting hormone replacement therapy (HRT) from natural sources.

I have to admit that I was nervous about starting treatment, especially since I'd heard about findings of the Women's Health Initiative (WHI), a research program established by the National Institutes of Health. More than 16,000 healthy postmenopausal American women who were between the ages of 50 and 79 and had their uteruses intact took part in the program, which was to last a number of years. Participants were daily given a placebo (sugar pill), or they were given a tablet of 0.625 mg of conjugated equine estrogen (that is, produced by horses) and 2.5 mg of medroxyprogesterone acetate (synthetic, *not* natural, progesterone). The study was designed to evaluate the use of synthetic HRT by healthy women for disease prevention, and good results were expected. But this was not the case.

Researchers halted the study prematurely because participants on synthetic equine HRT exceeded the boundary for breast-cancer risk that was established at the beginning of the project, and they were also at an increased risk for heart disease compared to the placebo group. The study further revealed that the women given HRT were at greater risk of strokes, memory loss, and fatal blood clots. As soon as these findings were released, women by the thousands panicked and threw out their hormones.

Since the WHI data had just been released, I felt a bit gun shy when my doctor recommended hormone therapy, but I had no reason to be personally alarmed. I'd never taken traditional HRT—I figured that because I wasn't a horse, my body didn't need it. My doctor allayed my fears, assuring me that with blood testing and frequent monitoring, the risks with bioidentical (that is, natural) hormone replacement therapy (BHRT) were minimal.

I went home to think about it, and that's when it hit me. A few months earlier, I'd been settling into bed at about 10 P.M. when I began to feel a strange sense of foreboding, and I sank down into a depressed state—which was very unusual for me. At the time, I'd wondered how the black hand of depression could be visiting me at a time when I was at my happiest. I was engaged to be married to a wonderful man, we'd just purchased a new home together, and my career was successful and fulfilling.

I now started to weep uncontrollably as I realized that what I'd felt hadn't been simply emotions . . . it was all about hormones. And I had another "aha moment" when I mused, *If this is how I'm feeling, and millions of other men and women are feeling the same way, then depression could be hormonally related.*

I knew that if my mood went unchecked, and I continued to spiral down into some black hole, my body would be open to a serious illness. The next thought came to me so strongly: *This is how a person could develop cancer.* I was open and laid bare, and if things continued this way, my immune system could become compromised—leaving an open door to cancer. What a thought.

The next day, I went back to my doctor's office and had all the necessary blood testing done. The results showed low levels of estrogen, progesterone, and testosterone. Based on the testing, my hormones would need to be balanced by taking natural estrogen; along with testosterone for increased energy, fat burning, sex drive, and sense of well-being; and progesterone for better bone building, sleep, and tranquility.

The moment I started taking natural hormones, I could feel the difference—this was it! Gone were the mood swings, the weepiness, the crabbiness, and the memory and weight issues. It's now four years later— I'm still using BHRT, and I've never felt better. I know that being on hormones is helping me slow down the aging process and feel happy and optimistic about my life. I'm so grateful to have learned about the value of hormones.

Natural vs. Synthetic Hormones

It really pays to know your hormones, as they're not all created equal—there's no "one size fits all" where the body's messengers are concerned. Hormones that are chemically identical to those found in the human body are called "natural," "human," or "bioidentical"; and they're made with plant-based or herbal formulas.

Such hormones are made in the laboratory via a process known as "Marker degradaton," which was originally discovered by chemist Russell Marker way back in the 1930s. He found that diosgenin in plant oils— usually from inexpensive sources, such as Mexican wild yam, which is not indigenous to Mexico and is actually more like a weed than a yam—can be subjected to chemicals that convert it into hormone components.

I find it interesting that since the publication of the WHI's findings, there has been a significant drop in breast- and uterine-cancer rates in the U.S. Could this be related to the fact that so many women have discontinued traditional HRT and are now investigating the bioidentical option?

There have been many articles published on BHRT to date, but it hasn't been scientifically researched yet. Despite the groundswell of women who are now seeking this therapy, it's remarkable that these naturally derived hormones have never been scientifically compared to conventional HRT. It's disturbing to think that plant-based hormones have been in existence for decades, yet they were then sidestepped. Luckily for us, they were rediscovered when they were vitally needed.

Synthetic hormones are manufactured with a chemical makeup that isn't found in the human body, but it does mimic some of the body's natural hormonal activity. These products are usually derived from the urine of pregnant horses. It's also worth noting that at one point a certain drug manufacturer wanted a progesterone-like substance that could be patented, as such a drug would obviously be more profitable than a natural hormone would be. Manufacturers supposedly started with progesterone and found ways to modify it so that it became medroxyprogesterone acetate, which could then be patented. This is not the same substance as natural progesterone . . . take it from me.

Years ago, a doctor prescribed medroxyprogesterone for me. I bloated up and felt terrible; after a month, I figured this was no way to feel, so I threw away the pills. Then when I revisited the whole hormone equation, I began to take natural progesterone, which was a much better choice.

I advise you to stay away from synthetic hormones— instead, use something that's a perfect match for your own body. Your symptoms, the way you feel, and your blood tests will determine the appropriate strategies and dosing used by your medical doctor or practitioner.

Bring on the Experts

In my seminars, we discuss the importance of hormones, and I try to steer participants toward the appropriate professionals to help them. As I tell these people, I know it can be difficult to find an expert to guide your hormone compass in the right direction. But if you put the "word" out to the universe that you'd like to connect with the best bioidentical hormone practitioner in your area, sure enough, a name will be presented to you in a very short time. That's the way the universe works—it delivers! You just have to pay attention to its signs.

Try asking your regular pharmacist for the name of a compounding pharmacy in your city. Such a pharmacy will be able to create bioidentical hormones for you; the preparations are "compounded" based on your symptoms, hormone levels, and blood work or saliva testing, which has been provided by your physician. Remember that the physician or practitioner prescribes the appropriate hormones for you, and then the compounding pharmacy creates your individualized prescription. In other words, compounded hormones can't be obtained without a doctor's prescription.

Another way to locate your nearest compounding pharmacy is to contact the International Academy of Compounding Pharmacists, which is a nonprofit organization representing pharmacies that compound custom hormones and other medications. If you log on to their

Website (**www.iacprx.org**) and enter your zip code, it will give you the name of a compounding pharmacy in your area. You can also call the toll-free referral line at (800) 927-4227.

After you've located a compounding pharmacy, call and ask for the name of the medical doctors or practitioners they work with. Remember that good news travels fast, so word of mouth is the best way to find a good practitioner.

I truly believe that the universe is always delivering information directly to me. Anything that I need—any reference, any contact, any piece of information, and any person to help me in my work or personal life—will be brought to me by the flow of life. In the case of hormones, this is exactly what has happened.

I started out with my family physician, who referred me to my Ob-gyn specialist. A family nurse practitioner introduced herself to me at a talk I gave. And finally, a doctor colleague of mine in Chicago introduced me to a font of information, Larry Frieders, R.Ph., who is the owner and compounding pharmacist of The Compounder in Aurora, Illinois (**www.thecompounder. com**). In fact, I was so impressed by Larry's knowledge of bioidentical hormones that I did hours of interviews with him and created a CD set to share with the rest of the world. (For more information, please see the listing of my products in the back of this book.)

I've also been blessed to have a wonderful association with Suzy Cohen, R.Ph., author of *The 24-Hour Pharmacist* (HarperCollins), who is very hormone savvy. Suzy's informative column about medications and complementary therapies appears weekly in many newspapers across the country, and it's probably the best collection of sensible health advice you'll find anywhere. (Please visit: **www.dearpharmacist.com**.)

Even with all of this support and information, I always rely on my gut instincts and the way I feel, and blood or saliva testing merely confirms my hunches. In Canada, saliva-testing kits may be ordered through **www.newmoonhealth.com**. If you're in the U.S., they can be purchased from Larry Frieder's Website, or from the following sources:

- ZRT Laboratory: **www.zrtlab.com**

- Women's International Pharmacy: **www.womensinternational.com**

- Dr. John Lee: **www.johnleemd.com**

- Virginia Hopkins Health Watch: **www.virginiahopkinstestkits.com**

Are You out of Balance?

Insulin is a master hormone, and this is the first part of balancing your hormones that doesn't require a doctor's prescription. If you're looking for a reference on ways to balance your hormones simply through diet and nutrition, *Dr. Susan Lark's Hormone Revolution* (Portola Press) offers many useful suggestions. (For more information, visit: **www.drlark.com**.)

However, you may not even know the common effects of hormone imbalance. Here they are, in no particular order (the symptoms listed tend to be felt by women, but men may have some of them, too):

— If your blood work or saliva testing shows that you're **estrogen deficient,** you could be experiencing hot flashes or night sweats, sleep-pattern interruptions, lack of sexual desire or painful intercourse, heart palpitations, bone-density loss, vaginal dryness, or depression.

— If your test shows that you have **excess estrogen,** you might be experiencing fluid retention or bloating, lumpy or tender breasts, uterine fibroids, heavy periods, yeast infections, fatigue, poor concentration, memory loss, anxiety, thinning hair, excess weight gain, endometriosis, severe premenstrual syndrome (PMS), low sex drive, or an elevated risk for uterine or breast cancer.

— **Testosterone deficiency** can lead to low energy, moodiness, lack of interest in life, memory loss, low libido, fatigue, and balance and focus problems.

— **Excess progesterone** contributes to the same symptoms as the excess estrogen listed above: fluid retention or bloating, lumpy or tender breasts, uterine fibroids, heavy periods, yeast infections, fatigue, poor concentration, memory loss, anxiety, thinning hair, excess weight gain, endometriosis, severe premenstrual syndrome (PMS), low sex drive, or an elevated risk for uterine or breast cancer. In addition, it can bring increased feelings of euphoria, crankiness, or irritability; drowsiness; and acne.

— Signs of **progesterone deficiency** are fluid retention or bloating, lumpy or tender breasts, fatigue, poor concentration or memory loss, thinning hair, excess weight gain, PMS, insomnia, or disturbed sleep patterns.

(**Note:** Postmenopausal women are most likely to be progesterone deficient, since this is the hormone that declines rapidly once menopause begins.)

Declining Hormones and Age

As we age, our body's reserves of hormones decline. Or, said another way, when hormone levels decline, we age. It's as simple as that.

If men notice that their hair has started to thin or turn gray, they've developed excess belly fat, they get tired when they're supposed to feel perky, their sex drive has become nonexistent, and they've become moody and grouchy, know that it has nothing to do with a dip in the stock market or the wintertime blues. These are signs of hormone imbalance.

Women are presented with another set of problems: It starts with the hot flashes—when, at any given moment, we break out in a sweat that sends rivers down to our underwear. Getting a good night's sleep becomes a critical issue that we never had before. We get these sudden heart palpitations that make us think that we're about to have a coronary on the spot. We discover that our bone-density scans have revealed that we have the beginnings of osteoporosis, which means that our bones are becoming more and more brittle; intercourse becomes painful (assuming we even feel like it); and a bout of tearfulness could hit at any time. And then we might start to notice memory lapses or find ourselves doing silly things, like putting the milk in the pantry and the crackers in the refrigerator! These new developments don't point to astrological or spiritual misalignments . . . again, they're signs of hormonal imbalance.

Fortunately, due to a great deal of new information—and the pioneering work of Suzanne Somers, whose book *Ageless: The Naked Truth about Bioidentical Hormones* (Crown) hit the mainstream media and made an intuitive "ding" with women everywhere—we are well ahead of the hormone hornet's nest. These days, women and men have a better chance than ever before of getting it right. We won't have to experience the decline we've seen in our parents, because now we have answers.

The next chapter looks more closely at those answers as they pertain to men and women, both together and separately.

CHAPTER 14

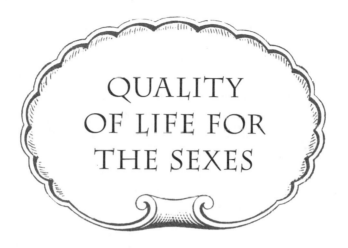

QUALITY
OF LIFE FOR
THE SEXES

After many years of being a single woman on my own, I'm now living with a man: my wonderful husband. I can attest to the fact that once his hormones were balanced, he got a whole new lease on life. Of course, underscoring his increased energy and well-being was a complete dietary change—lowering his starch and sugar consumption balanced out his insulin levels. But hormones were the icing on the cake, and I'm happy about that!

While women may think that they're the only ones going through hormonal changes, men go through them, too. In fact, anti-aging specialists say that an increasing number of their patients are men, and this is a very exciting trend. We should *all* be seeking perfect endocrine balance, as both men and women want to feel good physically and emotionally. We'd like to be calm, stable, and balanced; with boundless energy, a strong libido, a great sense of well-being, and zest for life throughout all of our days.

This is absolutely possible, for there are many medical doctors, practitioners, and experts whose expertise is devoted to balancing hormones for both men and women. Take Joe Filbeck, M.D., for example. Dr. Filbeck is the medical director of the Palm La Jolla Medical Spa in San Diego and an expert in healthy aging who specializes in a field called "quality of life" medicine. I love that term, since it reflects what we're all trying to improve.

I had a chance to interview Dr. Filbeck when he was an exciting presenter at one of my conferences, and I found that his interest in quality-of-life medicine began because Alzheimer's disease runs in his family. As he said, "I got into this work to save my own brain!" Formerly an anesthesiologist in conventional medicine, Dr. Filbeck realized 15 years ago that there were strategies for preventing chronic degenerative disease that were worth pursuing.

Dr. Filbeck finds the interest in vibrant aging by laypeople and professionals really encouraging, as this is the wave of the future. His patient base is comprised of about 40 percent men, who are keenly interested in bioidentical hormone balancing, testosterone, and HGH therapy as part of their vibrant-aging program. He finds this work the most fulfilling chapter in his career as a physician, telling me, "Disease can be turned around . . . people can get their lives back." (Please visit: **www. palmlajolla.com**.)

Let's take a look at some male-oriented concerns first.

Special Challenges for Men

When men develop a midlife paunch or become moody, grumpy, sleepy, or forgetful, then hormone balancing is worth investigating. Testosterone levels in men decline 10 percent each decade, starting when they're in their 30s. Then warning lights begin to flash, and all the symptoms of andropause, or male menopause, kick in.

Suzanne Somers's book *Ageless* offers valuable information on male menopause as well as sound interviews with leading physicians who are working in this fascinating field. Her book points to the fact that both men's and women's hope for an optimistic future is dependent on lifestyle changes and balanced hormones.

My primary-care physician also specializes in male menopause. As hormone levels decline, he believes that testosterone and DHEA help to restore a man's vitality, energy, muscle mass, libido, bone health, and well-being. When we discussed the controversial human growth hormone as a therapy, he did not recommend it. But other anti-aging specialists are very positive about it—one of them I know has been taking it for 25 years!

Prostate cancer is another concern for men, particularly as its rates are on the rise: In 2007, according to the National Cancer Institute, there were about 220,000 prostate-cancer diagnoses and 27,000 deaths. I'm intuitively aware that there must be a relationship between prostate cancer and elevated levels of estrogen, largely a result of our high-starch, high-sugar diets. Many men are also big meat eaters, and unless they're organic, most meats are laden with injected hormones. So the combination of these increased estrogen levels and declining testosterone levels are a likely explanation for prostate problems in men.

Studies have revealed that high or normal testosterone levels show minimal prostate enlargement, and that
high estrogen levels are more likely the link to prostate
enlargement. After all, if elevated testosterone caused
prostate cancer, then wouldn't we see cancer in 18-year-
olds instead of in men in their 60s and older? Sometimes
this concept is viewed skeptically by medical practitioners . . . maybe it's just too logical.

In support of the theory of testosterone being prostate protective, Eugene Shippen, M.D. (along with William Fryer), has written an outstanding book, *The Testosterone Syndrome: The Critical Factor for Energy, Health,
& Sexuality—Reversing the Male Menopause* (M. Evans and
Company). In it, Dr. Shippen points out that testosterone deficiency affects every cell and sinew in the body.
He describes it as a "thief in the night that robs a man of
his ambition, energy, and sexual drive."

Why does it take so long for sound ideas such as
those of Dr. Shippen to penetrate the bastions of mainstream medicine? It baffles me why the obvious continually seems to be overlooked. There's a great line in the
Bible: "[A]nd a little child shall lead them" (Isaiah 11:6).
Where's the wisdom and inquisitiveness of the child
who will lead us out of these medical mazes? It seems
that we'll have to decipher them for ourselves.

Another health recommendation for men to follow is examining their scrotum about once a week to
check for lumps, hard spots, or abnormalities that could
be indicative of a cancerous condition. And my family

physician, the male-menopause expert, says that men can protect themselves from prostate cancer by ensuring that testosterone levels are adequate and not too low. Rising estrogen levels and declining testosterone levels in men contribute to memory loss, low sex drive, lack of muscle strength, breast development, and the rounded physical frame that resembles that of a female. Your doctor can test your testosterone levels—when they're replaced at optimal levels, this increases sexual function, brain function, and performance.

Surprisingly, progesterone is another hormone that can be deficient in men, especially if they're eating estrogen-laden foods and exposing themselves to other sources of the hormone, such as dry-cleaning chemicals, plasticizers, or pesticides. Progesterone is involved in brain function, prostate protection, and sexual performance. I've read that as men age, they benefit from a daily application of 8 to 12 mg progesterone cream to the scrotum. The good news is that a little dab on the "crown jewels" can extend the duration of an erection.

When it comes to women in the sexual-gratification department, a small amount of testosterone cream applied to the clitoris 20 minutes before intercourse can heighten orgasm. That tip was given to me by Dr. Theresa Ramsey, a wonderful naturopathic physician from Scottsdale, Arizona, and the author of *Healing 101: A Guide to Creating the Foundation for Complete Wellness* (Center for Natural Healing Press). (Please visit: **www. drramsey.com.**)

Ingrid and Marnie

The world of medical intuition is fascinating. When I look into a physical body, I see it in terms of the systems that are out of balance. When I intuitively read a crowd of people, there are very few who aren't hormonally out of balance: If there's a weight problem, that's a hormone imbalance; if they're tired, that's a hormone imbalance (usually thyroid); if I sense memory troubles, that's generally thanks to a yeast overgrowth *and* a hormone imbalance. When men experience grouchiness and moodiness, that can be a hormone imbalance, too.

Sadly, many people are looking in the wrong place to determine the cause of their emotional issues. They blame themselves and their past decisions for their mental angst, when it may actually stem from an endocrine imbalance (which is one of the most commonly imbalanced systems in the body). This is completely correctable, and here are two stories to illustrate my point:

— Ingrid and I have been friends for years, and she's now in her mid-70s. The other day she called to say that she hadn't been well lately and had been spiraling down into depression. I was aware that she'd been on hormones and looking and feeling younger than her years. But then her doctor advised her to greatly reduce her hormones (probably because of the results of the Women's Health Initiative study I mentioned in the last chapter), and that's when her problems started.

I knew that Ingrid was suffering from a hormone imbalance, so I advised her to read some of the latest information about natural balancing and to get a blood panel done. I also urged her to encourage her doctor to put her back on her full complement of hormones—hopefully bioidentical.

I was greatly upset that my friend had been given the typical line of treatment for the aging female, and it resulted in a serious quality-of-life issue for her. Thankfully, she now had the tools to get back on track.

— Marnie had been referred to me by a fellow author who felt that there might be a physical reason for her emotional troubles. This 63-year-old woman was experiencing anxiety, depression, memory loss, and bone-density issues that had her very worried. She'd also consulted several healers and psychics, all of whom pointed to her troubling emotional past and anomalies in her astrological chart.

I took one look at her photo and determined through the sound of her voice that her issues had nothing whatsoever to do with astrology—this was a classic case of hormonal imbalance. Now, two practitioners and three months later, she's sleeping better, her memory has returned, and she's feeling like her old self. I was so sorry that she'd had to spend needless hours and countless dollars consulting with people who had no understanding of her postmenopausal condition.

A Woman's Chapters

The process of menopause actually contains several chapters, including premenopause, perimenopause, and postmenopause. During all of these chapters, changes are constantly taking place in our bodies, and they can be very confusing. Basically, what happens is that our master endocrine glands and reproductive organs operate differently, and their functions slow down. Even though we may be missing body parts, such as our ovaries or uterus, our endocrine system is still functioning (albeit not in a balanced or youthful manner).

As we age, our desire and focus should be to encourage these glands to function optimally in the most natural way, which can be accomplished with diet, nutritional supplements, and bioidentical hormone compounds. This is a delicate balance, but it can be achieved—and our well-being as we age depends on it. If it's warranted, the addition of estrogen, progesterone, testosterone, and DHEA (and, for some people, HGH) can make a measurable difference to our quality of life.

Most women believe that when they stop bleeding, menopause is over and the whole issue can be forever forgotten. Wrong. If we're going to be proactive about vibrant aging, then hormones need to be balanced for the rest of our lives, regardless of the cessation of menses. In fact, when I started reading books about bioidentical hormone replacement therapy (BHRT), several of them mentioned a protocol for natural hormone balancing that included cycling or having a monthly period. I was a little disturbed at the thought of having to stock pads and tampons again, after having given all that up at the age of 57 when I had my last period. As far-fetched as this might seem, one of the books even described an 82-year-old woman who still had periods!

Many doctors feel that this approach is much too radical, yet some practitioners favor cycling because it's deemed to be protective of the uterus. Continuous BHRT can contribute to a buildup of the uterine lining if the balance isn't correct, causing too much estrogen to be present. Initiating a monthly period can prevent this from happening.

I had several discussions with my primary-care physician and my ob-gyn about this, and they both said that cycling wasn't necessary—but I instinctively felt that it was. So for five days each month, I don't take my compounded hormones, and then I have a very light period that lasts about two days. This is an individual choice, and one that you'd need to discuss with your own doctor.

I know that my emotional and physical well-being have been greatly enhanced by the addition of bioidentical hormone balancing. I suggest that you get more information, get yourself tested, and start on this path to vibrant aging. This kind of help could have prevented a lifetime of misery for a dear friend of mine.

Janika and I have been close for years, and our children grew up together. She was a capable active-investment dealer with a bright, happy attitude . . . that is, until her first child, Cindy, was born. Janika went through postpartum depression and was so distant from her new baby that her parents had to move in and manage the household. My friend was put on antidepressant medication, and things eventually returned to normal. She also made weekly visits to a psychiatrist to delve into a past that, by most accounts, was normal and happy.

Years later, a light shone on Janika's situation that made perfect sense. Her doctor prescribed BHRT for her menopause symptoms, giving her a prescription for a mild dose of estrogen and progesterone cream to bring up her very low levels. All of a sudden, Janika felt like her old self, something that had eluded her for 34 years. When we talked over lunch a few weeks ago, she told me that she realized her postpartum depression all those years ago was probably related to low progesterone, not an "antidepressant deficiency."

If you know of anyone suffering from postpartum depression, please encourage her to be tested for hormonal imbalances, most notably low progesterone. Progesterone levels plummet following the birth of a baby—thus bringing on the "baby blues," which sometimes don't go away. And while progesterone is a very important part of the hormone chain, so is estrogen.

Estrogen Dominance

A common imbalance for both women and men is what Dr. John Lee, one of the pioneers of natural hormone balancing, called "estrogen dominance." This is what happens when estrogen levels are greater than the body's ability to produce adequate progesterone, thus creating an imbalance.

An important value calculated by saliva testing is the progesterone-to-estradiol ratio: Estrogen levels may be normal, or even low, but if progesterone is deficient, the person will experience symptoms associated with estrogen dominance. The key is the amount of progesterone, which can often appear low in menopausal women in relationship to estrogen. In fact, progesterone levels fall much more rapidly than those of estrogen do as a woman enters hormonal decline.

Compounding pharmacists say that the estrogen-to-progesterone level is alarmingly high in many women because of poor diets and the absorption of environmental estrogens. So we can thank our excess carbohydrate consumption from sugars and starches in the diet; hormone-injected meats; "estrogen mimickers" that we ingest through chemicals, pesticides, plastics, or estrogen-loaded dairy products; medications such as birth control pills; or synthetic hormone replacement therapy (HRT)—these substances all act like estrogen in the body.

Because of this endocrine imbalance, weight gain can start to build up during midlife, and people who lack consistent exercise can easily develop estrogen dominance. Omentum—a band of fatty, estrogen-loaded tissue—hangs like an apron around the waist. This excess tissue is a physical demonstration of estrogen dominance, and men are just as likely to spread out in middle age as their female counterparts are.

Estrogen dominance and that pesky spare tire around your middle may seem insurmountable, but high levels of the hormone can be balanced with diet and progesterone, and symptoms (which may also include weepiness, anxiety, cravings for starches and sugars, poor concentration, depression, fatigue, decreased libido, bleeding issues, spotting, heavy periods, bloating, and insomnia) will usually subside. Always work with your practitioner to achieve the correct balance.

Soy and Estrogen Dominance

If you're having trouble losing weight or you have enduring digestive problems, you might want to decrease your soy intake. You may recall that soy is a common allergen because of its indigestibility (it's a bean). Soy is associated with endocrine imbalances, and it can increase estrogen activity by "tricking" the body into thinking that it doesn't need to make as much—and low measured levels are actually one of the ways that people display estrogen-dominant symptoms. Soy can suppress thyroid function and block the absorption of iron and B vitamins, and it's been implicated in reduced sperm counts and poor libido in men. One of my Japanese clients even told me that her mother used to feed her father soy when she didn't want to have sex that night.

The Western body is not designed to assimilate soy, for it's simply not part of our food heritage. A study done on Japanese women showed that they experienced very few menopausal symptoms as a result of their soy consumption. When that study was then dumped on Western women, who weren't predisposed to tolerate soy, it evidently backfired. Only men and women whose cultures have used soy for thousands of years can tolerate it.

It's also important to keep in mind that almost all of the Asian soy studies are related to fermented products, not the actual bean itself. It was a leap in logic to connect fermented soy with soy protein and say that they're equal, when they are not. Tempe and miso, for instance, are fermented sources of soy and therefore may be more digestible.

A very useful reference for understanding this subject is *The Whole Soy Story: The Dark Side of America's Favorite Health Food,* by Kaayla T. Daniel, Ph.D., CCN (New Trends Publishing). This book is a devastating indictment of the safety of soy foods and how they can disrupt hormone function, not just in adults, but in children as well. Several years ago I used to refer many of my clients to a medical doctor in Arizona for hormone balancing, and I remember his concern even then. "Caroline," he said, "I can foresee an epidemic increase in breast cancer as a result of the pervasive use of soy in so many foods."

Women, Hormones, and the Risk of Cancer

If you're like me, the word *cancer* can be very scary, especially if you're taking hormones (even natural ones). I'm very proactive about hormone testing: I have a blood test and a saliva test done for all my hormones each year. I'm also sure to have a pelvic ultrasound and a mammogram done annually.

I know that cancer in most cases is an age-related disease, and that hormones can protect us against it. Last year I happened to be perusing a publisher's Website when I came across a book that caught my attention. I must have been ready for the next step! *Safe Estrogen: Reduce Your Breast Cancer Risk by 90%* (Vitality Press), by Dr. Edward Conley, provided me with an important piece of information about breast cancer prevention and estrogen testing. This is a very well-written and researched book that outlines several important strategies for reducing the risk of cancer.

If you're a woman, you may be aware of breast- and endometrial-cancer risks, but perhaps you're not familiar with preventive strategies. If you go to Dr. Conley's Website (**www.cfids.com**), you can order a test called the Estrogen Metabolite Index (EMI) to determine how well your body is detoxifying estrogen. This simple urine test is one of the best predictors of your breast-cancer risk, as someone with a low EMI is apparently more at risk than someone with a higher index is.

Dr. Conley also provides strategies to improve your test levels, such as supporting and cleansing your liver to promote the detoxification of estrogen. He also recommends taking specific supplements, such as diindolylmethane (DIM), which comes from broccoli and cauliflower and directs the breakdown of estrogen, thus reducing cancer risk.

You can also protect yourself by regularly drinking green tea; eating turmeric, flaxseed, and cruciferous vegetables; minimizing exposure to plastics that contain xenoestrogens; and building up your immune system by taking antioxidants and reducing stress.

Hormones and Bone Loss

As soon as women threw out their synthetic hormones after the WHI study, traditional HRT sales plummeted, and drug companies lost millions of dollars. So, in order to recoup these losses, advertising for various bone-density prescriptions hit the airwaves. These drugs claimed to build bone density and prevent more than a million fractures per year.

According to statistics, more than 30 million Americans either have osteoporosis or are at risk for the crippling condition. But medications to treat it come with side effects such as heartburn, chest pain, difficulty breathing, or stomach problems—and they can actually burn holes in the esophagus! I took one look at the side effects of these drugs and knew that I wouldn't be taking them.

Some people have even developed bone loss in the jaw as a result of using these medications. Symptoms include jaw pain, loose teeth, gum infection, or a slow healing following dental surgery. My friend Donna, for instance, is now waiting to have three tooth implants as a result of taking osteoporosis drugs for the past ten years. And a flight attendant I met who took them was told by two dentists to discontinue their use right away or her jawbone "would turn to chalk." I know of one dental office that's unwilling to remove teeth from people who have taken these medications because healing is interrupted (I was told of one woman who has a spot in her mouth that remains unhealed after several years).

According to dentists, the jaw area seems to respond quickly to the negative effects of osteoporosis drugs. The same thing happens to other bones in the body—they may appear to be dense on an x-ray, but they're really just "chalk." Bone is a living material, while chalk is compressed dead materials. Bone can heal; broken chalk remains just that.

The chemicals used in this group of drugs contain bisphosphonates, the same chemicals that have traditionally been used in the textile and fertilizer industries to prevent corrosion. When added to osteoporosis medications, those chemicals are designed to alter the cycle of bone formation and breakdown in the body.

Bisphosphonates also interfere with normal estrogen and progesterone activity and are considered to be hormone disrupters. Estrogen stimulates the normal breakdown of bone, while progesterone stimulates bone replacement, and that's how broken bones knit back together again. The drugs in question interrupt this activity.

There's a prescription nasal spray available called Miacalcin that's been shown to increase bone density without side effects. It has the same chemical makeup as the hormone a salmon produces to create its spine, known as calcitonin. Studies have shown that in fish, rodents, and some domestic animals, this hormone appears to play a significant role in calcium balance.

What Will They Think of Next?

Now that women are wary of synthetic HRT and osteoporosis medications, the latest word is that drug companies are planning to market an antidepressant drug to take care of sleep problems, night sweats, and hot flashes. *Please exercise caution here.* Menopausal symptoms aren't related to an antidepressant deficiency; these are hormone-related issues. Bone loss indicates declining levels of estrogen and progesterone—so weight-bearing exercise, absorbable calcium, a good diet, supplementation, vitamin D, and digestive enzymes all play a vital role in keeping bones healthy and strong.

On the subject of calcium, advertising would have us believe that drinking milk is good for our bones. This is not necessarily so: Sweden, a country with the highest dairy-product consumption, also has the highest incidence of osteoporosis.

Metaphysical Hormone Correlations

I'd like to close this chapter on hormonal balancing for the sexes by taking a look at testosterone deficiency and estrogen dominance on another level. There seems to be a higher metaphysical reason for male hormonal imbalances: Women are becoming more assertive, dominant, and capable in the world—they're not just content to sit at home and raise babies anymore. Could this be a direct cultural reflection of an estrogen-dominant society, where women become aggressive, while males become passive? After all, high levels of progesterone can make a woman feel calm, happy, and content . . .

the perfect environment for pregnancy and child rearing. Interesting!

On a subconscious level, men today may feel overpowered and dominated by women, thus contributing to a level of emasculation. Moreover, traditional gender roles are being redefined and may result in sexuality-related imbalances and diseases, commonly of the prostate.

Estrogen notwithstanding, women have fought for their equal position in all facets of professional life. So could it also be that spiritually speaking, it's time for women to have more of an influence in the affairs of our currently male-dominated world? It's something to think about. . . .

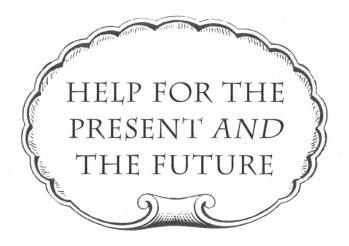

CHAPTER 15

HELP FOR THE PRESENT *AND* THE FUTURE

* *

Dr. John R. Lee and co-author Virginia Hopkins spell out the hormone story in their very informative book *What Your Doctor May Not Tell You about Menopause: The Breakthrough Book on Natural Hormone Balance* (Warner Books). Reading books like this, learning how your body works, understanding the rise and fall of your hormone cycles, and being familiar with the history of hormone replacement therapy and menopause politics provides you with the information to make informed decisions about your body now and in the future.

And although a well-known drug company that manufactures synthetic hormones would like you to believe otherwise, hormone balancing is not just a temporary program. These messengers in your body are continually fluctuating, so adjustments and refinements will need to be made along the way.

This chapter will help you understand how important it is to keep your hormones balanced . . . all throughout your life.

A Good Night's Sleep

The "sleep that knits up the ravell'd sleave of care," as Shakespeare wrote, can be elusive as we age. That's because the sleep pattern that we took for granted when we were younger starts to starts to change as we enter our 50s.

I know many people who get into bed dog tired, shut their eyes, and try to get the rest they desperately need, but to no avail. It seems as though the snoring spouse, the barking dog, and the ticking clock down the hall are right inside their ears. What's going on?

If you're menopausal, estrogen dominance can lead to anxiety, nervousness, and insomnia. While many people tell me that their "inner guidance" wakes them up in the middle of the night to meditate or write a chapter in their book, their sleep interruption is probably more related to hormones.

Ask your doctor to test your progesterone levels, which may be low in relationship to estrogen. When taken at bedtime, progesterone has a calming, relaxing effect on the body. You can also discuss melatonin supplementation with him or her and ask to have your level tested. Melatonin is a hormone secreted by the pineal gland that's involved in sleep-cycle regulation, and its levels decline as we age.

I'm lucky in that I don't have any trouble sleeping. When my head touches the pillow, I'm out. No matter what's happening in my life, even if I'm under some type of stress or pressure, I sleep like a baby. I'm also a firm believer in a hot bath before bed. At 9:30 P.M., I'm running my bathwater, ready for my half-hour soak—this, combined with a cup of chamomile tea, helps me sleep deeply.

Aging and Weight Gain

One of the biggest issues that women (and men) complain about as they get older is the inability to lose weight. Metabolic changes, declining hormone levels, and estrogen dominance can make weight loss a challenge . . . but I hope this story will inspire you.

I just happened to be working at home one particular day when the phone rang. Something made me pick it up (not a usual occurrence), and I was introduced to Mimi. It seems that she'd been struggling with obesity for many years and had almost given up hope But then, like a miracle, the book that would change her life was placed in her hands: A friend had picked up *The Body "Knows"* at a Hay House conference and given it to Mimi to read.

Here's what this remarkable woman says about her lifelong battle with excess weight:

> I've had a weight problem since I was 13 years old. I've tried every type of diet out there, and all of them ended up in failure. When I took a trip to Paris with my family a few years ago, I weighed 350 pounds. With this kind of weight problem, I'd been living in my own little world, existing within a small circle between my work and home. The trip to France posed

new challenges and brought me face-to-face with my weight issues.

On July 18th, 2005, at the age of 55, I made the decision that I'd had enough. After barely being able to fit into an airplane seat and having great difficulty keeping up with my family in Paris, the severe pain in my massive body and my lack of energy and self-esteem just made me say, "This is it!" With tears of anguish pouring down my face in that Paris hotel, I made the decision to give up everything I loved—ice cream, garlic bread, mashed potatoes, and chocolate. I figured that had to be the key . . . and lo and behold, the weight started to come off.

Three months later, a friend gave me Caroline Sutherland's book. I realized that the program I'd been following was exactly what was outlined in it, only I didn't know why it had been working. *The Body "Knows,"* and the food plan contained within its pages, brought me the missing pieces: Finally, here were the explanations for why I'd experienced a lifetime of cravings; and why food allergies, yeast, and hormone imbalances were the root of my problems. Following this program has liberated me from food, and it's given me back my power and self-esteem. I feel good about myself.

A huge part of my success comes from listening to a special CD that Caroline created, called *Why Wait to Lose Weight?* Listening to this CD has helped me change my attitude and rescript my mind, which I like to do as I work on one of my favorite crafts, beadwork. Rescripting my mind on a daily basis keeps me on track and motivated toward my goal weight of 160 pounds. I know I can do it, especially since I've already lost 125 pounds. I'm ecstatic!

These are some of my successes:

- I can now fit into a chair with arms, I can tie my shoes and squat down, and I can get up from the floor without crawling. I no longer have pain in my back and legs, and I can even cross my legs for the first time in many years!

- I used to have to go to bed as soon as I came home from work because I was so exhausted. Now I have boundless energy and can go out with my friends—I even took a cruise. Also, my blood pressure has returned to normal.

- I had to go out and buy a whole new wardrobe, which I'll have to do again when I lose another 50 pounds. Last week, I bought a pair of pants with a zipper instead of an elastic waistband . . . that's a first!

- When I took baths, I used to put six inches of water in the tub, but it would then be full after I added my body. Now I can put 18 inches of water in, and fit into the tub very comfortably.

All these things are breakthroughs for me. They may seem small to you, but to a very overweight person, they're huge milestones. And if I can lose weight, you certainly can.

The universe got the information to Mimi at the right time because she was ready. Thus, the guidelines and suggestions in my book made sense to her.

One of the qualities she also possessed was determination. She saw the results reflected in her body as soon as she started the program; she knew that she was experiencing a miracle, and she was bound and determined to keep going. This is something about Mimi that continues to impress me. Plus, she's an inspiration to many others: She works in a health-food store, speaking to hundreds of people each week who are encouraged by her success and the way she looks. She's found her purpose by uplifting and educating others, and this helps her stay on track with her own health goals.

Why did Mimi gain weight to begin with? Well, why does anyone gain excessive pounds? Usually, it's because they're using food to satisfy a void in their lives, or to fill up the deep hole within the little boy or girl inside. Mimi was able to get back in touch with her own body and reconnect with that person inside—the real Mimi. She was committed to her program and the progress she was making, and in the process, she discovered that she could teach and motivate others. She could understand their situation from personal experience, and now she's become a catalyst to change lives.

Weight-Loss Strategies

In order to lose weight, you need to understand that there are five key components that must be paid attention to in order for you to be successful. We've covered all of these elements in depth in this book, but here's a brief recap:

1. Most overweight people have **food allergies** or sensitivities, often to the things they consume every day.

When they eat offending foods, they puff up and gain weight as a result of histamine reactions.

2. Overweight men and women tend to be afflicted with an overgrowth of **Candida yeast**, which can create tremendous cravings for starches and sugars that can seem out of control. The Candida-yeast syndrome is easy to correct with supplementation and diet.

3. **Carbohydrates** convert quickly to sugar, and excess sugar is stored in the fat cells. Carb grams should be lowered to about 60 per day, most of which ought to be derived from vegetables.

4. The body is designed to move, so **exercise!** Stimulate your lymphatic system, tune and tone up muscles and fibers, increase your heart rate, and oxygenate your brain. Choose something simple that you can commit to every day, such as swimming, walking, Pilates, yoga, or some other mild exercise routine.

5. Probably the biggest component of the weight question as we age is **hormones.** Middle-aged people who are overweight often have thyroid and related endocrine problems. For women, menopause is a time when we have a tendency to put on extra pounds, which can be so frustrating, especially when many of us aren't overeating!

Hormones require careful balancing, so if that's not done, successful weight loss may be elusive. In fact, if you've tried food-allergy avoidance, limiting carbohydrate grams, controlling yeast, and exercising daily, but you've reached a plateau in your quest for the ideal body weight, this usually points to a hormone imbalance.

When it comes to hormones and weight gain, don't blame yourself for what's happened—it's not your attitude, history, or emotional problems that are at fault here. Seek help from a competent practitioner, and get the tests you need to start down the road to recovery. And remember that hormones are as individual as people, so what's good for Jane isn't necessarily good for Joan.

Looking at this issue more closely, the following two hormones are especially troublesome when it comes to weight gain:

— Menopausal women often find themselves putting on the pounds for no apparent reason, but it's actually thanks to the relative increase in **estrogen** compared to progesterone, as I mentioned earlier. Imbalanced levels of this hormone can also contribute to cellulite—yes, that ugly, lumpy material on thighs and buttocks is the result of a decline in estrogen, which starts between the ages of 25 and 35.

My research in hormone imbalances led me to the wonderful work of Dr. Lionel Bissoon, author of *The Cellulite Cure* (Meso Press). According to Dr. Bissoon, when estrogen levels decrease, several things happen: Blood vessels become smaller in diameter, as well as harder and more fibrous, and they decrease in number. Once this happens, the collagen fibers that give our skin elasticity and integrity, and that also surround fat cells, become weakened. Then these fat cells enlarge and herniate (or rupture) the collagen fibers, leading to visible cellulite.

Once this sequence of events is initiated, it becomes a vicious cycle: With a decrease in oxygen supply to thigh and buttock tissue because of weakened blood vessels, toxic waste builds up, and free-radical formation leads to continuous cellulite formation.

Dr. Bissoon says that this sequence of events not only happens in the thighs, but throughout the entire body. Because there are estrogen receptors in all tissues, many women start to show signs of aging in their 30s; as they approach menopause, these symptoms will increase because of the gradual decline in the body's own estrogen production. Dr. Bissoon recommends BHRT early in a woman's life.

Here's another little tip: You'll notice a lot less cellulite if you avoid dairy products and caffeine. These two items affect the lymph system, and toxic buildup in the lymph contributes to cellulite.

— Another reason why midlife pounds can be hard to shed can be found in the **cortisol** equation. Cortisol is a steroid hormone that's produced in the adrenal glands and is often referred to as the "stress hormone," since it's released when we become stressed . . . and how often does that happen?! An imbalance of cortisol can increase blood-pressure and blood-sugar levels, and it can suppress your immune system.

Too much cortisol—from prolonged stress, as well as too much insulin in the blood—affects adrenal function and creates fatigue, irritability, and metabolic imbalances and weight gain. High cortisol levels can particularly contribute to excess padding around the waist, which can be nigh impossible to get rid of. Increased levels can also contribute to adrenal exhaustion, causing you to feel really tired. Saliva or blood testing can determine cortisol levels.

A Lifetime of Work in Progress

We need to be aware that as women and men in midlife, we're constantly changing on an endocrine level. So unless hormones are balanced, carbohydrate grams are counted, and an exercise plan is instituted, we won't achieve the levels of vitality and well-being that we're seeking.

Because cycles and symptoms are always changing, in order to achieve hormone balance, you should be working with your practitioner on a regular basis throughout your life. You should be in it for the long term.

Yes, hormone compounds cost money, but I consider them a necessity, just like all my other household expenditures. I'm happy to pay the price for the way I feel, and it's a given that I'll be balancing hormones for the next 30 years or more. I look to my neighbor Vi, who at age 90 has been taking them (although not bioidentical ones) for the past 20 years, and she's going strong.

You'll know when your hormones need to be checked by the way you feel: You should have great energy, glowing skin, a clear mind, and optimism and vitality. Throw in a wonderful libido, and you have the equation for eternal youth! If you're not feeling this way, then the hormone compounds you're taking need to change—even a subtle difference in the way you feel is a reason to go back to your doctor for an adjustment. Your symptoms, plus saliva or blood tests, will determine a new course of action.

Some hormone compounds cause side effects, so do know what they are. There's no need to settle for weight gain and feeling awful—keep researching and asking questions.

I believe that the future for men and women lies in specifically tailored hormone compounds, which are calibrated on an individual basis to match each person's changing endocrine system. I also believe that it's worth every cent and every bit of energy we have to get our hormones balanced. As the years go by, our quality of life will be largely dependent on maintaining a healthy diet and lifestyle, as well as youthful hormone levels.

This didn't make sense to a woman who piped up at a recent presentation I gave at a bookstore. "Why should I do anything that defies gravity, nature, or the course of events that my body seems to be on?" she asked "If I'm aging and declining, why should I slow down that process with hormones?"

I told her it's for the simple reason that if we're living longer, we could endure up to 30 years of declining health. Who wants that? Certainly not me! I also let her know that there are many studies that demonstrate the benefits of estrogen replacement, for instance, which include increased collagen production, skin elasticity, and circulation; as well as a decrease in the number of wrinkles. My aesthetician tells me that she can always tell by looking at a woman's skin if she's taking estrogen or other hormones.

However, not everyone needs hormones. Unlike Suzanne Somers, who advocates their use for all women, I think it's wiser to approach them with conservative, professional direction and use them *only if needed* to balance your individual needs. For example, I know a lady who's 73 and looks and feels terrific, so she sees no need for hormones. Sure, she carries a little extra weight around her belly, but her skin is clear and youthful, and her memory is sharp.

Hormone balancing should always be a personal choice, as everyone is different.

Now, in the final section of this book, I'm going to address the final secret of vibrant aging: igniting passion.

PART IV

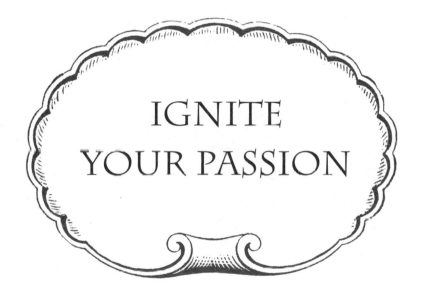

IGNITE
YOUR PASSION

CHAPTER 16

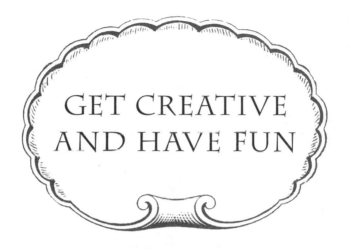

GET CREATIVE
AND HAVE FUN

. . . .

The fourth and final step in the vibrant-aging equation is to ignite your passion. Before you read any further, I want you to take a moment to evaluate how engaged you feel with life. After getting out a piece of paper and a pen, find a peaceful place in your home and take a few deep breaths. As you inhale and exhale deeply and center yourself, know that all of the answers to your questions reside within.

Put your hand on your heart and access your inner wisdom. Ask yourself, *How fast am I aging? Would it be at a 20 percent or 50 percent rate? Or am I totally aging at 100 percent?* I want you to get a specific figure—if you just stay quiet, the answer will come to you. (When I tune into my own body, I get an aging rate of 30 percent, which means that 70 percent of my body is regenerating and repairing.) Jot down the number you receive.

Now think about what you can do to slow down your aging rate: Might it be through changing your diet, exercising more frequently, lowering your stress, or simplifying your life? Write down the answers you receive.

Next, with your hand back on your heart, ask yourself, *What is my personal level of happiness on a scale of one to ten?* Wait for the answer to come . . . it could be a surprise. You may think you're totally happy, but your heart knows that something is missing. If that's the case, then this chapter will especially resonate with you.

Loving Life

When asked, "What gets you out of bed?" a couple of elderly friends of mine chirped in unison, "When we need to get up and pee!" Well, every morning I get out of bed somewhere between 5:00 and 6:00, and peeing is not my motivation—I'm ready and excited to get on with life. I'm on fire with passion, commitment, and excitement because I get to help others improve the quality of their lives.

When people ask me how I get my energy, I tell them it's from following all the guidelines I've outlined in these pages so far. If *you* enjoy a healthy diet; remove poisons and allergens from your body and mind; and support your body with lifestyle changes, supplementation, and bioidentical hormones (if necessary), you'll have boundless energy and mental clarity, too.

In this book, I've addressed the physical components of healthy aging—detoxification, rejuvenation, and hormone balancing—and without them, the final element is probably going to be elusive. We need energy, vitality, and stamina to execute our soul's purpose; in other words, it takes all of the elements that I've written about in this book to keep this passion alive.

When you can see the way forward, the universe can use you, and your soul can complete its destiny. Your soul or inner compass speaks to you all the time, telling you, *This feels right . . . I like how this sounds . . . I feel like doing this . . . I don't feel like going there . . . I'm attracted to this . . . this makes sense to me,* and so on. You become disconnected from your inner compass when you're weighed down by the toxins, addictions, and burdens of life—when no lightness, optimism, or balance can reach you. Loving life and enjoying yourself will help you hear your soul's messages again.

So in order to light your fire and stay fully alive and engaged for the rest of your days, you're going to have to increase your "fun quotient." Having fun rates very high on my list of ways to ignite my passion. I'm passionate about my work, but I'm just as passionate about play. I do what makes me happy, even if it may seem childish.

I grew up in a large old house right by the ocean in the Pacific Northwest. On the front lawn, hitched onto a branch of a huge maple tree, was a swing—it had such long ropes that I could swing way up in the sky, which was magic for a child. In our spare time, my siblings and I would all run to see who could get on it first, and sometimes my sister and I would stand up and swing together. This was quite an adventure, considering that if either one of us fell off, we'd land in a huge patch of prickly bramble bushes below. I have many fond memories of hours spent on this swing.

Enjoying a swing has been important for me in low times as well as high. I remember when I went through my divorce many years ago and my life was completely turned upside down. There was a school near my home, and early in the morning I'd walk over to it and spend time on one of the swings. And even though I'm 64 and happily married now, I still can't resist a swing.

At this stage in life, we can follow our heart's desire and have the freedom to do what we want regardless of people's opinions. For example, at almost 70 years of age, Kate injects fun and adventure into her life every day of the year . . . and she's also a little eccentric. She's an ocean swimmer, even in the winter, and for years her morning routine has been to ride her bicycle down a steep hill to the beach. Rain or shine, she then disrobes down to her "birthday suit" and takes a quick dip in the (sometimes frigid) water. Then she dries off, puts on a warm sweat suit, picks up a few pieces of driftwood that she puts into her bike's basket, and pedals home.

I encountered another such individual last summer. My husband and I had taken a daylong trip on an interisland ferryboat in beautiful British Columbia, and we were getting off to have lunch on one of the islands. As we were disembarking, I looked over to see an older woman putting on a helmet and getting on a bright red motor scooter. She was quite a sight: She had a healthy, ruddy complexion that she didn't cover up with makeup, and she wore a T-shirt that said "ARIZONA GUARD DOG" underneath a picture of a rattlesnake.

There she was, boobs down to her navel, wearing baggy shorts and funky shoes, but clearly having fun. She told me that she was in her 70s but rode her scooter everywhere, and on this particular day, she was going to see her doctor on a neighboring island. She didn't much care what she looked like or what anyone thought—she was enjoying life and having fun. All I could think was: *Bravo to you!*

Sex and Passion

Speaking of fun, sex can be a beautiful form of expression between two people, no matter how old they are. In fact, a 2004 study by the AARP (formerly the American Association of Retired Persons) showed that a healthy percentage of people age 65 and over enjoy sexual activity at least once a week. It seems that in our later years, we feel more relaxed, have a better understanding of the nature of giving, and aren't as self-conscious about our bodies. So what if it's all hanging out (or down)—chances are our partner's body is in the same state, and the bonus is that he or she probably can't see that closely without glasses! In all seriousness, having sex with someone we deeply care about is quite a bonding experience. And as love grows between two people, intimacy acts can be more pleasurable and satisfying.

In my seminars and presentations, I'm always quick to point out that people should be on the alert for their sexual passions to be rekindled after following a program of yeast eradication, dietary changes, and hormone balancing. And I tell them, "If you don't have a partner, then you might consider purchasing one and keeping it in the bottom drawer, since you'll probably be calling on it!" A reawakened libido is very exciting, for it means that the body is in good health. Even better than that, it's returning to its natural youthful vibrancy—which is something to rejoice about.

Sexual activity should absolutely be enjoyed in our later years, as it helps us feel in touch with the beat or pulse of life. While of course it's earthy and physical, it can also be very spiritual and healing. The Tibetans say that there are two states that generate an abundance of energy: one is anger, and the other is sex. They believe that if properly channeled, sex becomes an offering and can raise one's spiritual vibration. On the other hand, anger is a powerful form of energy that needs to be mastered and brought under control. That is to say, one passion needs to be tamed, the other ignited.

Unlocking the Creative Genius

There is a creative genius within each of us that's just waiting to be born—it can even be reached through meditation when we get in touch with our higher teacher. That's what happened to me back in 1988 when I went with a friend to see Bernie Siegel, the well-known medical doctor who wrote the famous book *Love, Medicine & Miracles: Lessons Learned about Self-Healing from a Surgeon's Experience with Exceptional Patients* (HarperCollins).

Dr. Siegel was a pioneer; a giant; and a much-needed voice in the body, mind, and spirit movement at that time. Hundreds of us had gathered in a large auditorium to hear him speak. After giving a very powerful and uplifting speech, he led us in a meditation in which he encouraged us to imagine that we were on a path by the edge of a river.

In my personal visualization, I could see myself sitting on a rock at the edge of this river, and I was painting.

A few tears sprang into my eyes, and I remember feeling very happy and peaceful. I came out of the meditation and told my friend that I'd been painting in it.

"Maybe you *are* going to paint," she mused.

"Me, paint? Why, I haven't done any artwork since high school," I retorted. "I can't imagine where I'd even begin."

"Well," said my friend, "you never know."

That was a Tuesday night. Two days later, on Thursday, I'd arranged to meet another friend for lunch. She lived in another part of town, and after we finished eating, she asked me to drive her to her painting class because her car was being serviced. When we got to the building, she wanted me to come in and meet the art teacher.

"Oh, I couldn't do that," I protested. "It would be too disruptive." Yet she begged me to come in, saying that the teacher was very spiritual and would love to meet me.

I reluctantly went into the classroom, met the teacher, and was promptly given a set of paints and brushes and asked to join the class. The rest is history: All my high school love of art (although I'd studied sculpture, not painting) came flooding back, and I had my first show several months later. I've been an inspired painter for many years now.

My creativity is inspired by my higher teacher, which we all have. This exercise, which calls on the four powers of personal creation, helps unlock the creative genius:

1. Power—the Mountain

I recently visited Tibet, where I was struck by the immense power of nature. Many elements of this book were actually given to me during meditations in which I connected to the power I felt there.

Bringing in the energy of power enables us to create plans and stay focused on them; we can also remove obstacles, which allows our destiny to move forward.

Breathe in the mountain; breathe out power.

2. Vastness—the Sky

I'm sure that you've experienced a place in your life where you were able to witness a clear, open sky—I was struck by such a sky in Tibet. In calling on this power of vastness and limitlessness, we open up to more of the potential within us. As we age, we can shut down the feeling of unlimited possibility, believing that there isn't enough time or that we're too old to accomplish anything beyond our daily existence.

Breathe in the sky; breathe out vastness.

3. Creativity—Nature

Using the strength of the mountain and the vastness of the sky, we now call on the power of nature's creativity. Nature is always creating: The flower blooms, the tree puts forth new shoots, and the bees work in their hive . . . so it is with us. The image of nature helps us manifest what we want in our lives in terms of our destiny, healing, and purpose. Or we can create in simple ways that improve our home or environment.

Breathe in nature; breathe out creativity.

4. Deep Peace—the Still Lake

In Tibet, there's a special lake that's located high up in the mountains beneath a canopy of rarified air. No one lives there, and there are no boats or signs stuck in the ground—it's just a huge body of water that's a deep emerald green. When I saw this lake, it seemed to represent the concept of inner peace, something that seems either more attainable or elusive as we age. As we bring the feeling of peace into our body, our creative gifts, skills, and talents become more accessible.

Breathe in the still lake; breathe out peace.

Identifying Your Skills and Talents

Returning to the sheet of paper you used at the beginning of this chapter, make a list of all the things you love to do, such as singing, crafts, being in nature, painting, caring for animals, gardening, tinkering with cars, playing golf, writing, and so forth. Jot down whatever you can think of.

When Heather did this exercise, she realized that she was happiest around babies. She loved them dearly, even though she was a single woman in her 40s who had never married or had children of her own. Something inside her told her that she needed to be around little ones, so she helped out with her nieces and nephews and read stories to boys and girls at the local library. Heather had a great rapport with children of all ages, especially babies—she had a special knack for holding and speaking to them. She decided to take a nursing course and thought she might work in a hospital. But a chance meeting with an administrator at an adoption agency changed her plans.

Heather instead underwent special training to become an interim foster parent for newborns awaiting adoption. Her dream had come true: To be with babies—to hold them and give them love and attention until the timing was right for new parents to get them—was indeed Heather's higher purpose.

Part of turning on your passion comes from doing something that you love every day. My husband, Gary, adored English cars as a young man, for instance, so many years ago he bought an old Morgan (an English car whose frame is made of wood). Gary spent countless hours working on his Morgan and brought it back to life. Soon he was driving it around and attracting attention, as interested people kept striking up conversations with him.

Before Gary knew it, other Morgan owners had become his firm friends, and he decided that he should start a group. He formed the Morgan Owners Group Northwest, which grew into a large-scale operation with barbecues, car rallies, and other social events. That group now has branches in cities in the northwestern United States and in Canada. My husband was even honored at a dinner for his contribution of bringing the love of these old cars—and joy and happiness—into so many people's lives.

Listening to, and Then Answering, a Calling

Timing is everything. Abby was 45 and had arrived at the point where her career in banking was no longer fulfilling—she needed a change, but to do what? She had some vacation time saved up, and her husband, Jim, suggested that she spend it by going to the beach (they lived two blocks away). He said that she should let the ocean speak to her, as perhaps nature would hold an answer to her question. So every day during that vacation, Abby would go down to the beach and sit on a special rock. She let the peace of the ocean quiet her mind, but nothing came. She'd end up returning home to report to her husband that she hadn't received any startling insights . . . just a nice time at the beach.

Jim kept encouraging his wife to go back, because he knew that something would eventually be revealed to her. Abby faithfully returned to the same rock day after day. After two weeks of this, she finally received one word: *teach*. It had taken that long for this woman to quiet her mind enough to receive a message from the universe.

Abby went back to her rock by the beach for another few days to see if she received the same message. Indeed, the word *teach* kept coming to her. This would be a huge step for her to take, but it felt exciting. Then fear and panic struck her heart: What if she quit her secure job at the bank and trained to become a teacher, only to find out that she didn't like it? What if listening to her inner wisdom was just plain wrong? What if she didn't get good grades? What if there were no teaching jobs for her after she graduated? What if she just couldn't do it?

Abby's fears were valid, but her instinct that education was a good move won out, so she took that huge step forward. While her husband was still working and could support her, Abby pursued her teaching degree—it was very challenging, but she dedicated herself to it and persevered. Her guidance proved to be correct, for she feels so happy and fulfilled as a fourth-grade teacher. This new career has served another purpose as well: Now that Jim is retired and on a pension, Abby's income helps the couple financially. And since teachers get great vacations, the two of them are free to enjoy travel as well.

Like Noah, who had to endure people laughing while he built that wooden boat, Abby's ark (that is, her soul's intention) is now floating along happily after a brief period of discomfort.

~ ~

We may not know what it is, but there's an unseen force guiding our lives. Some of us recognize a need and respond to it, no matter what it takes or what our circumstances are, and we often don't know when we're going to be called to action. This brings to mind an amazing story of a truly extraordinary human being.

Father Alexander Tkachenko, a Russian priest, didn't wait for the right timing or financial circumstances to propel him into action. In 2003, he was a priest at St. Nicholas Cathedral when he was shocked to hear of the plight of terminally ill children in St. Petersburg. It seems that when medical treatment no longer provided hope of recovery, hospitals tended to send these boys and girls home to die—usually to a communal apartment. Families regularly shunned the children out of fear that their disease, which was frequently cancer, could somehow be transmitted to them; thus, the kids remained virtual prisoners in one room for many months, with few visitors and little hope.

Because the law in Russia required that strong painkillers only be given by injection, and because the doctor or nurse capable of administering the injections rarely did so, these poor souls were left to suffer in unmitigated pain. Then, after they died, their parents often divorced due to unbearable grief.

Father Alexander felt called upon to do something about this grave situation, so he organized a small group of doctors and nurses to assist these children. His effort was the birth of St. Petersburg Children's Hospice, the first of its kind in the history of Russia. The idea of a children's hospice in St. Petersburg actually had its genesis at a chaplains' training that Father Alexander attended at the Swedish Medical Center in Seattle. Because of that course, the seeds of Father Alexander's destiny were planted.

At first, Father Alexander relied on sister churches in St. Petersburg for support, but then through a series of fortuitous meetings, some churches and secular organizations in Seattle heard about his mission, and funding started to roll in. During his frequent trips from Russia, he spoke to these churches and other groups about his dream for the hospice. Word spread, and the project began to touch hearts all over the West, as well as back in St. Petersburg—where, fortunately, there's now more focus on the plight of dying young people. Their care is currently home or hospital based, but Father Alexander's vision is that one day there will be a facility in St. Petersburg to equal Canuck Place Children's Hospice in Vancouver, British Columbia, perhaps the finest children's hospice in the world.

THE BODY KNOWS . . .

Just like Father Alexander, maybe you know of a similar situation in your own community. When God wants a job done, He/She sends in the legions of support, so bring in the angels! If you're looking for ideas for yourself as an individual, I suggest that you read *Three Cups of Tea: One Man's Mission to Promote Peace . . . One School at a Time,* an uplifting story by Greg Mortenson and David Oliver Relin (Penguin). There's always an area for you to serve: You could be a mentor, for instance, taking a child under your wing and preventing him or her from experiencing the pitfalls of life.

Remember, you're an important thread in the tapestry of life's grand design. If you let these stories inspire you and you follow the guidelines I've given you in this book, you'll have the energy and vitality to leave your own soul imprint and do the work you were destined to do. It's your time. Call on the four personal attributes of power, vastness, creativity, and deep peace; and align with the Great Spirit to complete your work on this planet.

Staying on Purpose

My passion is helping people and seeing them reach their highest potential, yet I had no idea that this was "it" until I turned 40 years old and attended my first meditation retreat. During a visualization process, I got in touch with my inner guidance, and a phrase came to me: *Your purpose is to motivate and help people.* At that point, it wasn't revealed that this purpose would be related to the field of integrative medicine. I just listened and followed my inner guidance and did what felt right to me at the time. My own ark is now floating—my purpose has fully manifested, as I was told it would be all those years ago.

Your purpose is to be all that you were intended to be, to reach your full potential before you die. Achieving this level of personal self-mastery means turning on your "destiny switch": Realize that it's your life, it's up to you, the time is now, and you're in control of everything in your world.

Most people think of life as a haphazard chain of events that just happen as they go along; they work at jobs they don't like and force themselves through their daily rituals with very little joy or fulfillment. This doesn't need to be you, and if you keep climbing to the summit of your personal mountain and moving toward your destiny, it won't be.

As Peggy McColl teaches, there's nothing more fulfilling than being on purpose. I met Peggy during the publicity campaign for my book *The Body "Knows" Diet: Cracking the Weight-Loss Code* and found that she's just like me—a woman living her destiny. In *Your Destiny Switch: Master Your Key Emotions, and Attract the Life of Your Dreams!* (Hay House), Peggy gives us important tools to take this last chapter in our lives and fill it with motivation and zest, making it a rich and experiential one. Of course emotions are going to come up, she says, but she teaches us how to replace those that judge or limit us with more positive attributes. Thus, by using courage, kindness, inspiration, wonder, and the like, we can reach our destiny.

We're Never Too Old

When I think of my life and all the wonderful things I still wish to do, I never feel too old. I'm not daunted by my physical age or any possible limitations. Sure, I'm a senior, but what I really feel like is a senior who's just finished high school—like I'm about to step out and make my mark on the world. I'm fully aware of my chronological age, yet I know that my true age is many years less.

There's lots of time to experience the wonders of life, especially if you listen to anti-aging experts, who are now saying that we can live well past 100. After all, a destiny path never stops leading us on. Even Albert Schweitzer, the famous doctor who started an African hospital for people afflicted with leprosy, talked about finding our true purpose. He suggested that this should be something that fills our whole life, takes all our attention, commands our spirit, and is never fully complete. As there are many never-ending rivers and tributaries that lead to a purpose, it will indeed keep growing, building, and changing. We stay passionate about our destiny for a lifetime.

Finding, and then committing to, a destiny path means accessing your spirituality at a deep core level, which brings us to the next chapter.

CHAPTER 17

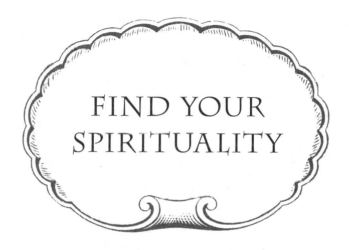

FIND YOUR SPIRITUALITY

. . . .

In the shadow of the Himalayas, including towering Mount Everest, lies the rugged country of Tibet. I had the opportunity to visit this place in the spring of 2007, and it was truly an inspiring experience.

I've always wanted to go to this country, and I was even compelled to paint a picture of it in 1986: Entitled *Tibetan Sunrise,* it hangs in my bedroom, and I look at it every day I'm at home. This painting reminds me that there are places in this world that are locations of spiritual power, no matter what goes on around them. To me, Tibet is one of the main anchor points for healing and peace that radiate out into the world on a daily basis.

Buddhism is alive and well in this country, despite politics and other challenges. If you ever feel down or depressed in your life, just know that thousands of

Tibetan people are praying, chanting, spinning their prayer wheels, and fingering their beads while doing their mantras—all for you! Buddhists pray for "all sentient beings," which means everyone everywhere, regardless of circumstances, alignments, or sentiments.

In fact, one of my favorite experiences during my visit to this incredible country was listening to monks and nuns chant in the monasteries and nunneries I visited. I was immediately drawn into their vibration of deep peace and power. The stunning artifacts, paintings, and wall hangings I saw didn't matter to me as much as the quality that emanated from the people living so simply within those walls. It was evident that Buddhism is a simple religion, and there's really no need for great cathedrals or any complicated philosophy.

In my observation, Tibetan people fully embody the principles of tolerance, living in the moment, deep appreciation, spirituality—and, above all else, an acceptance of things as they are despite the odds. These are qualities that all of us should seek to embody ourselves.

I was also extremely attracted to the land—I continually wanted to be outside, connecting to the power of those high mountains and what they were trying to tell me. "Lift your spirits, let go, and remove old patterns of limitation. Let the immense power of the universe fill your body and soul," they seemed to say.

Basking in the energy of the Tibetan peaks, I felt the vibration, essence, and purity of my surroundings—from the rugged land beneath to the expansive sky above—and something moved within me. During my entire two-week visit, I could feel Mount Everest's energy channeling through me and clearing the way for this book to be written. It was an awesome experience, and in the next few pages, I'd like to share the insights I received with you.

Harnessing Power Through Meditation

Meditation is vitally important to a healthy-aging plan, and it works best when done from a power center. (**Note:** Never meditate while driving!) Create such a spot in your own home: It could be an entire room, a corner of your office or bedroom, or a simple chair that faces a window. It's preferable that your power center looks out into nature.

If you don't have a mountain or hill to gaze upon from your power center, locate a picture of your favorite peak (mine is Mount Everest, or what the Tibetans call "Qomolangma," which means "Mother"). Are you particularly drawn to Mount Fuji; Mount Kilimanjaro; Mount Popocatepetl; or one of the Cascades, such as Mount Rainier in Washington, Mount Hood in Oregon, or Mount Shasta in California?

After you've found an image you like, concentrate on it for a few minutes. Now you're ready for the following meditation, in which you're going to use that mountain to unleash your own personal power and potential. (You may want to read it into a tape recorder first, and then play it back when you're ready.)

> *Sit in a comfortable position and close your eyes. Take a deep breath in, hold it for a few seconds, and then let it out. Take another deep breath in, hold it for another few seconds, and let it out. Take a third deep breath in, hold it for a few seconds again, but this time let it out slowly.*

Imagine your mountain: It is towering, powerful, and covered with snow; yet it is close enough for you to feel its presence and its energy. As you focus on this image, keep taking deep breaths. You are going to breathe in the energy of the mountain and then let it go out into the world:

Breathe in power; breathe out strength.

Breathe in might and solidity; breathe out release.

Breathe in stability and confidence; breathe out unlimited potential.

Breathe in magnitude and presence; breathe out poise.

Continue to do this as many times as you like.

Next, think of an obstacle, be it a person, place, situation, or thing. Now feel the energy and power of the mountain—in front of you, behind you, and within you—blasting through that obstacle and making the way clear again. Once again, take some deep breaths as you visualize yourself solving this problem:

Breathe in clarity and unlimited power; breathe out a clear path.

Breathe in peace and acceptance; breathe out self-realization.

Breathe in possibility; breathe out limitlessness.

Again, continue to do this as many times as you like.

Finally, ask the quality of the mountain to dissolve all blocks that exist within <u>you,</u> thus returning the power of the mountain to you.

If you take just a few minutes each day to practice this meditation, in a few days or weeks you'll see many positive changes in your life.

The Four Alignments

As I've already mentioned, passion on all levels keeps us young and healthy. But year after year, as I look out over the seas of people I see in my classes and seminars, I can tell that so many of them are far removed from their true calling. I can intuitively feel that they're not on purpose, and this lack of spiritual alignment is where disease begins.

If you feel this way yourself, what can you do to align spiritually? I find that there are forces that can orient your inner compass toward your true purpose—I call them "the four alignments," and they're powerful spiritual figures who represent the qualities of power, wisdom, love, and peace. While I use Moses, Buddha, Jesus Christ, and the Virgin Mary, please feel free to choose your own examples who feel right for *you*. Be sure to pick those individuals whom you'll feel comfortable using as training models to follow, as you aspire to reach your highest potential.

1. Moses—Power

You may remember the Old Testament story of Moses; if not, allow me to refresh your memory.

When the future prophet was a baby, his mother put him in a basket in the Nile River so that he wouldn't be killed because of his Hebrew heritage. Soon the basket floated downstream and was picked up by the Pharaoh's family, who raised him as their own.

After Moses had grown up and become very involved in Egyptian life and the mistreatment of slaves, he learned of his humble origins. When he sided with other members of his tribe, this did not bode well with the authorities of the day, so he fled Egypt and became a shepherd.

Many years later, Moses was sitting up in the hills quietly tending his sheep, when he looked over to see a small bush that had spontaneously caught on fire. (This famous account of Moses and the burning bush is probably read in Christian churches and Jewish synagogues at least once a year all around the world.)

Moses stared at the bush in disbelief, and then he heard a voice calling to him over and over again—it was directing him to free the Hebrews from their Egyptian captors. Moses felt that surely God had made a mistake, since by this time he was an old man. Yet the voice kept repeating that this was what he was supposed to do, so that old man reluctantly set off for Egypt, not knowing how he'd accomplish the daunting task that had been asked of him.

When Moses arrived back in his homeland, he formed a plan to set the slaves free, and he was aided by several plagues that mightily tormented the country. When the Pharaoh grudgingly agreed to finally let the Hebrews go, Moses led them out into the desert in the middle of the night. By the time morning arrived, the slaves' absence had stirred up quite a bit of anger among their former captors.

When Moses and his group found themselves at the edge of the Red Sea with nowhere to go, and Egyptian

soldiers in chariots gaining on them, they became panicked. That's when, in a desperate and bold move, Moses
commanded the waters to part. They did indeed, and
Moses and his followers were able to make it safely to the
other side before the sea came back together, drowning
the Egyptian pursuers in the process.

What does this mean symbolically? Well, let's start
with the burning bush, which is symbolic of our own
lives. Each one of us has had an experience when, all of
a sudden, the voice of wisdom spoke to us. Like Moses,
we probably weren't sure where the guidance came
from, although it did seem to originate from a higher
place that was unknown yet familiar, and something
compelled us to listen. It may have seemed scary at
first, but when we did as our inner guidance suggested,
it worked out. This is the voice of intuition that we're
called to follow.

Now, turning to the Red Sea story, we have all of its
elements within us. The Red Sea represents the obstacles
and blocks that prevent us from moving forward. The
captives are the parts of our mind that don't want to be
liberated from our self-made inner prisons. And Moses
is the leader within us, driving us forward to complete
our destiny. In order to get the job done and live our
soul's purpose, we need to call upon Moses and command these obstacles to move. (This can be done with
the power meditation I described a few pages back.)

When I almost died in 1995, I had a deep and powerful conversation with the Divine. I was told that it didn't
really matter what we looked like, what the quality of

our clothing was, or how much money we had—or even if we were healthy. What truly mattered was the quality of our hearts and the acts of loving service that we perform while we're alive. It was an awesome experience that has stayed with me, daily keeping me on track with my higher purpose. Even as we get older, we always have time to turn our lives around and focus on what our hearts are telling us.

2. Buddha—Wisdom

The concepts of Buddhism have interested me for many years. As my husband is a Buddhist, I'm now able to more deeply study some of the aspects of this spiritual discipline and integrate them into my own life. One of them shows up in the second alignment: wisdom.

During my trip to Tibet, I had the opportunity to see many people practice compassion and deep wisdom on a daily basis. It's ingrained in their spiritual tradition to be wise, understanding, and compassionate, despite all that they've endured.

Buddha was a great and powerful spiritual teacher from ancient India who apparently received his enlightened wisdom while sitting under the famous Bodhi tree. Also known as "Shakyamuni" or "Gautama," to Buddhists around the world, he is the revered Supreme Buddha of all time. He's believed to have lived about 500 years before the birth of Christ, and his spiritual discourses (which form the backbone of the Buddhist tradition) were originally passed down through an oral tradition. Decades later, they were committed to writing, and these ancient texts still survive to this day.

These are the Four Noble Truths, the core of the Buddhist religion:

- Life means suffering.

- The origin of suffering is attachment.

- The cessation of suffering is attainable.

- The path to the cessation of suffering is non-attachment.

Suffering is divided into three categories called "The Three Mental Poisons," which are central to Tibetan medicine. These can lead to various disorders, as follows:

- Acquisitiveness and greed—nervous-system disorders

- Anger and hatred—cardiovascular problems or cancer

- Self-deception and ignorance—digestive issues or mental disorders

The solution and end to suffering, according to the Tibetans, is to let go of the ego, attachment, and mental angst; while this may be easier said than done, it is the key to vibrant aging. Then the cravings, ignorance, and delusions are said to disappear as one progresses on the spiritual path—a lofty ideal that we can all aspire to. To have this knowledge that our own suffering begins in our minds and perceptions liberates us to embody the second alignment.

A Buddha (not to be confused with *the* Buddha) is someone who has become fully awakened to the truth; that is, the individual is enlightened to the extent that he or she has experienced nirvana or the heights of spiritual bliss and oneness. A Buddha possesses many important spiritual attributes, such as knowing, leadership, teaching, enlightenment, blessedness, worthiness, and personal mastery; and he or she has left the attachment of an ego-driven life behind. Such a person carries an energy or essence that's palpable or felt by others, becoming a great teacher. Teachers are necessary to point the way for others, who might not find the spiritual path on their own.

A Buddha teaches an understanding of the nature of suffering—that it's the result of the mind. All Buddhist traditions embrace the concept that a true Buddha has completely purified his or her mind of desire, aversion, and ignorance; in so doing, he or she is no longer bound by suffering and the dualistic nature of this world. We can all strive to achieve our own Buddha nature, particularly since wisdom is something that tends to be gained with age.

3. Christ—Love

The great spiritual master Jesus Christ represents the third alignment because, for many people around the world, he's the ultimate example of unconditional love. His message, just like that of the Buddha, is one that we can all aspire to. I'm more interested in the message than the man himself, and many times in my life, I've wondered, *What would Christ do here?*

Questions such as *Can I love this person or this situation? Can I forgive and move on?* and *Can I be like Jesus and accept someone who has betrayed me or let me down?* are lofty concepts that the Christ figure teaches us. However, keep in mind that Jesus wasn't all peaches and cream or love and happiness; according to biblical teachings, he had many tests and challenges and was known to buck the system, especially when he turned over the tables of the money changers in the temple. He also spoke up for the downtrodden and accepted women and minorities as equals.

I believe that Jesus was able to deal with the deeply troubling issues of his time because he believed that "I and the Father are one"(John 10:30). That meant that he and the Divine (what he called "the Father," I call "the Divine") cleaved together, thus forming an incredible partnership that was able to move mountains. I believe that forming our own partnership with the Divine or our inner guidance is the most important way to get in touch with, and then fully execute, our soul's purpose.

These are all concepts that we can see being played out in our own lives on a daily basis. Someone who brings this idea of love and acceptance into a daily perspective is a woman I greatly admire: Byron Katie, the author (with Stephen Mitchell) of *Loving What Is: Four*

Questions That Can Change Your Life (Random House). Katie explains that our suffering often comes from trying to change others, when we really need to change our own way of thinking. As a matter of fact, she says that we can end all suffering if we love and accept "what is," or the present reality of our situation.

Katie went through many years of depression and despair, only to wake up one morning filled with joy in the knowledge that what she was going through was of her own making—that is, her own misconceptions were keeping her stuck and miserable. Since that time, she's traveled the world teaching the principles of what she calls "The Work." I've seen her in action a number of times, and what she teaches is nothing short of miraculous. (Check out **www.thework.org**, and find out for yourself.)

4. Mary—Peace

The fourth alignment comes in the form of Mary, the ultimate representation of peace. The mother of Christ is one of the most revered figures in the Roman Catholic tradition: "Hail Mary, full of grace," is said at the beginning of the rosary, for example. I'm not Catholic (I was actually raised Episcopalian), but I've called upon the presence of Mary many times in my life.

Mary—a young woman who, by most accounts, never expected that she'd be asked to do anything more than live a simple existence—was suddenly thrust into the spotlight when an angel appeared to her. (A visitation from an angel would be pretty exceptional!) The angel told this unmarried virgin that she'd have a child

. . . and not just any child. Mary's baby would eventually impact the world and the course of history in a major way. This would have been a shock for anyone but Mary, who apparently took it all in stride and realized that she was part of a great plan.

Mary bore her child and became a peaceful, loving mother who only thought of nurturing the future King of Israel. She then watched her beloved boy grow up, move away from her, become a high spiritual teacher, and die a violent death at a very young age. Yet even as she was torn in anguish, Mary continued to be peaceful and loving.

Now, you may wonder who could possibly live up to these standards. Who could bear to witness the murder of her only child and still have peace and love in her heart? This is a tall order, and almost impossible for anyone to endure. But you're not meant to compare yourself to the mother of Jesus; rather, use her example to bring you peace. Whenever I'm sad or afraid, for instance, I call upon her presence. I can sense her peaceful essence surrounding me, to the point that I can almost feel her blue cape enveloping me. This helps me remain calm and comforted when no serenity is at hand.

As I've shared with you, I never felt the peace and comfort of a mother when I was a child. While it's interesting that my mom's name was also Mary, the bosom of my physical mother was no place to turn to. The energy of the Divine Mother replaced what I longed for growing up.

Mary also represents the mother within us who gives birth to our own Christ child—our personal soul creation or Divine purpose. As we progress on our soul path, her peace, love, and nurturing aids in bringing our purpose to fruition. By daily nurturing ourselves just like a mother would, we evolve spiritually and bring our gifts into the world.

Finally, the mythical figure of Mary is that presence of peace that we can bring into our own lives at any time—she's a model for how we can relate to others when communication might be difficult. When we're in a discordant situation, we can call upon her harmonious essence.

Climbing to Greater Heights

Each one of the four alignments of power, wisdom, love, and peace leads to a waking-up process that's so exciting. Aligning yourself with these four spiritual masters (or any spiritual presence you feel drawn to), allows you to evolve into your own best self. It's like peeling off the layers of an onion, one by one, to reveal the real you. I also believe that by working on the physical body, emotional and spiritual transformations take place more easily—through the process, you'll access your own personal worth and value.

It's constantly apparent to me that optimal health and well-being depend upon feeling cherished or supported, as lack of personal worth and value take the body's energy down. Always do your best to surround yourself with loving, helpful men and women. If you have people in your life who aren't such positive influences, know that they're likely trying to bring you down to make themselves feel better.

Yet we also draw individuals and experiences to us that directly reflect how we feel: Life is a mirror, so what's going on *within* us brings exactly the same thing *to* us. When we allow others to treat us poorly, it's because they're reflecting how we feel about ourselves.

When it comes to health, we use foods, substances, and addictive behaviors to cover up for the fact that we've lost touch with our self-worth . . . and then we get sick. If we emanate a low level of energy, then we're going to attract low energy to us, including people who aren't supportive or interested in improving themselves. We ultimately need to let go of these folks, which can be difficult and takes courage. The silver lining is that as we progress along on the spiritual path, we'll become less likely to attract anyone who's negative into our life.

As you climb your mountain of self-mastery, call upon the masters of the four spiritual alignments for help with any challenges you encounter. Also, try using "I am," which is the great power phrase: Say, "I am powerful," "I am capable," "I am love," "I am wise," "I am infinite in possibilities," and so on. The more you repeat this, the more you'll begin to feel that way. Rescripting what's inside of you will almost immediately be reflected in what's outside of you.

Years ago, I created a CD called *Letting Go of the Past & Moving Forward,* which was designed to help people in the transformational process. This CD can help you stay motivated while undergoing such significant changes, or the "dark night of the soul." Another potent and highly effective tool for this process is Bach Rescue Remedy. Bach Flower Essences were created years ago by a medical doctor in England, and each flower has a correlation to the emotions you're personally experiencing.

I suggest that you become familiar with these remedies, which are available at your local health-food store. At the height of my own transformational process, I must have downed quarts of Rescue Remedy, as it was an oasis of calm in a crazy world.

A daily meditation; any of the books, CDs, and healing products available from Hay House; and a brisk walk or connection with nature will help you transform as well. And remember that in the end, you'll heal your soul and bring out the person you're destined to become—fully alive.

Now let's delve deeper into the mysteries of transformation.

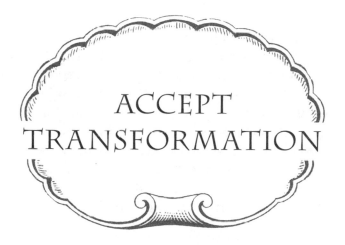

CHAPTER 18

ACCEPT TRANSFORMATION

· ·

While this may seem like an odd topic in a section on igniting your passion, it's hard to talk about living without also mentioning dying.

I saw my first dead body about 20 years ago as I was walking along the beach. I was shocked to see that, not 15 yards away from where I stood, a young woman had washed up on the shore. Her purse and clothes had been neatly placed in a pile on the sand, as if she were ready and prepared to end it all. (Indeed, the police later confirmed that the cause of death was suicide by drowning.) Yet this women seemed far too young to die.

The second dead body I saw was my 87-year-old mother, who died four years after suffering a ravaging stroke. She, on the other hand, had lived life to the fullest.

We in the modern world seem to be removed from death, but at the turn of the century this wasn't the case.

It wasn't unusual for families to lose a child to illness, a mother to childbirth, or a father to a farm injury—death was part of life.

These days, things are much different. Of course we're living longer, but since elderly people aren't part of the average household, death has also been removed to the outer fringes of our existence. Most of us have grown accustomed to not being as "up close and personal" with loved ones passing on as humans were in days gone by. However, I feel that our sense of removal from this important part of the life cycle shortchanges us. There is much we can learn from the transition we'll all ultimately make from this world to the next.

The Lessons of Living and Dying

While the end of life is inevitable for everyone, many of us in the West aren't prepared for it—instead, we're actively in denial when it comes to this subject. Contrast that with the Buddhist tradition, which teaches that no one can fully live until he or she addresses the subject of death. Tibetan Buddhists believe that we can't die peacefully if our lives have been consumed by violence, or if our mental state is overcome by fear, anger, or attachment. So experienced practitioners and spiritual masters (including the Dalai Lama himself) frequently acquaint themselves with the death process in meditation.

I recommend the *Tibetan Book of Living and Dying* (HarperCollins) by Sogyal Rinpoche, a renowned teacher of Tibetan Buddhism. This important book gives great insight into the Tibetan tradition of life and death, the nature of karma and rebirth, care of the dying, and the challenges and rewards of the spiritual path.

A Potent Symbol

I have a dramatic painting in my home that depicts an aspect of spirituality that few can accomplish.

In Tibetan Buddhism, there is an advanced spiritual practice wherein accomplished practitioners can actually bring their lives to a stunning and triumphant close. They've evolved beyond the dualistic grasping and ego-based existence, and they can transcend the normal process of death through a technique that they've perfected throughout their lives.

At the moment of their passing from this plane into the next, these enlightened ones are able to be absorbed back into the state of oneness from whence they came. Their physical shells dissolve into light and then totally disappear, a process called the "rainbow body" or body of light.

There are stories about the destruction of many temples and monasteries in Tibet where, when the aggressors arrived, all that was left of the monks were piles of clothes. They'd all dissolved into their rainbow bodies . . . and rainbows were also seen in the sky above.

Past Lives

If we wish to die well, then we must live well, too. The cycle of birth and rebirth is central to Buddhist teachings: They believe that the level of consciousness at the time of our death can directly influence the quality of our next birth, and that a virtuous state of mind in our daily lives and at our death will determine the outcome of our next life.

I've had very strong memories of past lives, which have come to me through meditation and visualization, as well as by taking workshops with skilled teachers. To that end, the work of Brian Weiss, M.D.—particularly his book *Many Lives, Many Masters: The True Story of a Prominent Psychiatrist, His Young Patient, and the Past-Life Therapy That Changed Both Their Lives* (Simon & Schuster)—can help you get in touch with your own past lives and how they might be impacting your current health and choices.

I once tapped into a life in China where I was a mother and a rice farmer, as well as the representative of the people in my village. One day we were visited by wealthy landowners who took our food and left us with nothing. My village's children were starving, and when I appealed to the landowners, a man held out a basket of rice to me. Just as I reached out to take it, he punched his fist through the bottom of the basket, scattering the grain in all directions on the ground.

In another incarnation, I was a servant in a wealthy home in Greece (a place I've always felt spiritually connected to). Once again, most of the poor people were starving; once again, I went to speak up to the authorities. This time I was admonished for my protestations and placed in a large wooden cage, through which I was fed only scraps. One night I got out and ran down to the waterfront, where I escaped in a small wooden boat. I rowed furiously out into the ocean, only to be engulfed by a severe storm and drowned. A third incarnation was more recent, when I died as an English soldier on the battlefield in France.

In the Buddhist tradition, it's believed that a soul is reincarnated and reborn over and over again until certain lessons are learned and the soul progresses. Therefore, we arrive on this planet not whole, perfect, and complete; but with a set of cells that contain emotional material that can predispose us to weak physical links that may appear later in life.

That brings me to my present life. First, let me paint a picture of what my mother was going through before I was born: The year was 1944, she was in her mid-30s, and she was about to give birth to her second child (me) without her husband. As this was smack-dab in the middle of World War II, my father, who was a ship's surgeon in the UK's Royal Navy, was aboard a destroyer in the middle of the Atlantic Ocean. Consequently, I believe that at the time of my birth, I was imprinted with deep patterns of worry, concern, and insecurity that have taken me a lifetime to overcome.

No matter what our history—in this lifetime or previous ones—to rise above, to gain strength, and to overcome limitations is our great quest. As we become more open and release these limitations, we can be more creative and open to letting love in . . . and that takes us to this book's final lesson.

CHAPTER 19

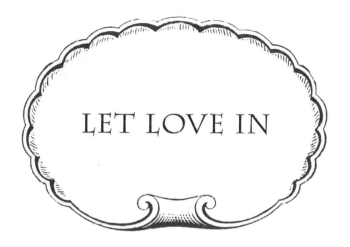

LET LOVE IN

Are you looking for love but wondering if the universe has forgotten about you? If so, don't give up. No matter how old you are, that special someone is destined to meet you when the time is right. Love is a powerful healer at any age, and certainly one of the best possible ways to ignite your passion.

If you need proof, I hope that the following story will give you all the evidence you need.

The Connection of a Lifetime

He walked into the room where I was teaching in Seattle on May 9, 2003. He was part of a group that had come from all parts of the country to this weekend seminar in order to learn how to become more intuitive about their own bodies, as well as those of their clients, family members, and friends.

Part of the training included an individual reading given by me, and as I sat down with this man, I sensed the death process. I knew that in five years he'd either be dead or very sick, as his will to live was almost nonexistent.

Whenever I sense that people are horribly off course, I try to engage them in conversation, grasping for a thread of what lights their fire. He told me, "My name is Gary, and I'm an oncology nurse." I stayed quiet and continued to listen within. When he added, "But that's all about to change," I thought, *Oh good.* Then he continued, "I'm going back to school to do my master's degree in nursing, and I'm going to be counseling cancer patients in the use of antidepressants."

Oh no, I thought, getting a sinking feeling. Yet I felt powerless to help him, since I had nothing to add—and the pressure was mounting to do readings for all the people still left in the room. "Well, at least it will be a change," I assured him, and then I handed him his completed reading.

Gary appeared to be enjoying himself over the course of the weekend, and at the end, he came up and gave me a hug. We said good-bye, and I never thought I'd see him again. However, I heard later that when he first saw me, a little voice inside his head said, *That's her!*

The universe was obviously orchestrating things on a higher level as about a month later, I had some presentations to give in Portland, Oregon, Gary's hometown. I had a chance meeting with Gary at a dinner for some of my dearest Portland friends—including June D'Estelle, my meditation teacher and the author of *The Illuminated Mind: A Step-by-Step Guide to Spiritual Discovery* (Alohem Press).

When I arrived at the restaurant, I couldn't believe my eyes. Gary had lost weight, and I no longer sensed the aura of death around him. The light of life was clearly so bright within him, and he looked energetic and vital . . . and very attractive. What a difference from the man I'd met the previous month in Seattle.

As my friends drove me back to my hotel later that evening, I remarked, "That man looked positively yummy—I could wrap him up and take him home!" Yet I truly didn't give the encounter another thought.

Then on July 15, *exactly* one month later, Gary turned up at a summer meditation retreat that I attend each year, although neither one of us knew that the other was going to be there. It was nice to see him, but I didn't pick up on anything else. However, we did happen to sit next to each other for several meditation cycles; and as I tuned in to him, I could sense that he was a sweet, dear man who exuded a wonderfully calm presence.

Gary had studied with a Buddhist lama for five years and is very knowledgeable about Buddhism in general, along with Tibet, its culture, and its spiritual practices. So when my friends who were hosting the retreat asked him to describe the symbolism of some of the Tibetan paintings that hung in their home, I found that I was very interested in what he had to say. As he spoke so eloquently about these works of art, I felt a strong connection to him. A spiritual giant was obviously in our midst.

Afterward, Gary showed us a very moving Buddhist spiritual practice, and we all gave him a big hug. I simply wanted to thank him for what he'd brought to the meditation retreat, and especially to my friends, who'd wondered about the meaning of their paintings for some time. He, however, had obviously picked up on something that I hadn't—at the end of the retreat, he asked for my phone number and e-mail address. He e-mailed or called me almost every day for more than a month, and then he decided to come visit me.

I must admit that I was a little apprehensive. I'd been on my own for 18 years and had built a rich, full life for myself. Even though from time to time I'd called out to the universe to bring that "special someone" into my life, I hadn't been lonely or pining. Nevertheless, it seemed that the gates of Fort Knox were about to be opened, and I was a nervous wreck! For the next five weeks, I existed solely on chicken soup, as nothing else would calm my stomach.

I kept thinking about something that had happened at the retreat. Over and over again, I passed a papier-mâché angel-wing art piece that was propped up against the wall at the bottom of a stairwell. Finally, on the last day of the retreat, I picked up the wing and asked one of my friends about it. She asked me if I'd like to take it home, and I said yes—for some reason, I felt that I needed to have this wing around me. When I got home and told her about Gary, she said, "Caroline, you've been flying on one wing for the past 18 years. Now Gary has come to be your other wing."

I knew that this man could be "him," and my life would be forever changed. Was I ready?

When Gary arrived for his four-day visit, the first thing he did was present me with a gift: a beautiful porcelain statue of Kuan-yin, the Buddhist deity of compassion. And things went very well from that point on—he even proposed to me within the first hour! We had a long, lingering kiss by the kitchen sink (if that condo is ever sold, the sink comes, too), and things progressed rapidly from there . . . we both just knew.

It turns out that Gary and I have so many things in common, including our shared interest in traditional and complementary medicine; our extensive spiritual research and practice; our love of theater, movies, travel, the outdoors, boating, food and cooking, current events, art, and history; and our passion for books, everything from Greek mythology to biographies. (He's extremely well read on many subjects.) There was so much for us to enjoy together.

I took Gary out on my boat and showed him the mountains, coves, and Howe Sound, where I've spent many happy hours. We visited a neighboring island for a meal and then traveled up to visit my daughter at her summer cabin, since I wanted at least one of my family members to meet him. We walked the seawall, went out for dinner, saw a play, and attended a service at my church—where, I'd later find out, Gary had an instant vision of our future marriage ceremony. Everything was magical.

Things went so smoothly, and we felt so compatible, that we felt as if we'd known each other forever. Then our visit came to an end, and Gary flew home. But as soon as he arrived, he checked his work schedule and saw a four-day window in which he was free and I could come visit him. I had the opportunity to see *his* world: to visit the Buddhist temple he attended, take a romantic walk through Portland's famous International Rose Test Garden, go out to dinner, visit the Columbia River, and even meet his parents!

Just a few months later, we bought a home together, and Gary presented me with a beautiful diamond ring the following New Year's Eve. We were married later that year on a pristine white beach in the Virgin Islands, and we honeymooned aboard a ship on a Caribbean cruise. This was followed by a church wedding—true to Gary's earlier vision—several months later, where we were surrounded by family and friends.

When Gary and I first met, he was 57 years old, and his lovely daughter was 19 and about to start college. He'd been married for 7 years and divorced for 12 . . . and then his ex-wife ended up dying of cancer on the very ward where he was the nurse in attendance. He is no stranger to pain and is surrounded by death and sick people in his work on a daily basis, but he's also cheerful and optimistic and doesn't appear to retain the energy of his surroundings. He must be like the Archangel Michael as he ministers to these sick people—he's a saint.

This man is a very nurturing person and a giver. After many years of my giving, giving, giving, it's so nice to be treated like a queen. My husband is a wonderful cook who also cleans up the kitchen right away and brings me tea. (Imagine having tea poured for you!) He's a consummate romantic, and his thoughtfulness is remarkable: He brings me flowers every week, opens the car door like a true gentleman, and puts the toilet seat down!

Like me, Gary is extremely intuitive, and he understands and is fascinated by my work and what it's all about. We have so much to share . . . and I have never felt so at home with anyone in my life.

The Lighthouse

Marriage has added a new and wonderful dimension to my world. Looking back on my single years, there's really no comparison. This is a love that covers my heart and soul, one that continues to grow and blossom as time goes by. And as I observe Gary in action, he helps me become a better person.

When he can, my husband accompanies me on my trips, and he's a fabulous help at seminars. As an oncology nurse, he's able to give his perspective on the deeper meaning of cancer, including why he believes people develop it in the first place; and he's knowledgeable, personable, and charming. Love at this stage is not hot and heavy (although it can be)—it's more like a warm blanket that covers me and heals up all the wounds of my life.

Gary and I have grown very close, and I can actually watch the progression of our relationship through the spiritual visions that I'm given from time to time. For example, the first night we made love and were lying in each other's arms, breathing quietly together, I was visited by a tall black angel who told me that he represented all the men who had been significant in my life. We stood on a white beach, and I could feel his large, warm hand place my own in Gary's; then Gary and I walked down the beach to a waiting rowboat. As we got in, the black angel gave me to Gary, and then he pushed the boat away from the shore—pushing me away from the past and into the future.

Gary rowed our boat toward a lighthouse in the distance, which was very bright and beckoning. In the next scene, I saw us in the lighthouse: He was reading or working at a table, while I was involved in the kitchen. We were together, but we weren't bonded at this stage of our relationship the way we are now.

I checked in frequently over the months, and each time I was given a new vision. I began to see us coming together as a couple—we might be in the lighthouse's kitchen, for instance, or both of us would be reading at the table. About a year into our relationship, things changed, and so did the vision: Gary and I were now dancing in the center of the lighthouse, happy and surrounded by light. To me, my marriage is a Divinely ordained relationship of two people destined to be together, sharing a common purpose, and surrounded by a circle of infinite love.

Manifesting That Special Person

I want to stress this point for you: *Don't give up on your belief that the right person is out there.* Prior to meeting Gary, I was single for a long time—while I'd met several nice men over the years, no one was permanent-commitment material. But when the time was right, events were quickly set into motion . . . and take it from me that the right person is worth the wait.

However, you can also manifest your soul mate. I actually did this about two years prior to meeting Gary: I started actively putting out the energy and the prayers to meet the right man for me. As I've already mentioned, I hadn't been pining for a partner, but I did want to experience that special relationship in my life. This all became very clear when I bought a boat for my birthday one year. As soon as I got my boat out on the ocean,

I knew that this was an experience that needed to be shared—I wanted to have someone sitting next to me to enjoy such a breathtaking experience.

I gave up on "lists" and specific traits and decided to simply turn the whole thing over to God, figuring that the Divine knew what was best for me. As I knew that energy draws things into our lives, the only visualization I settled on was sensing into the essence of this ideal man's being. I imagined him holding me in his arms, and I could feel his breath on my face. I felt his presence next to me without any particular definition, but I knew that he had blonde hair, blue eyes, and a very boyish face with soft, clean-shaven cheeks. But most important, I felt his beautiful heart.

All of the above is exactly what I have manifested! God has presented me with the physical form of my soul mate, identical to my vision. I feel blessed, happy, peaceful, and content in Gary's presence . . . how could I be this lucky?

An interesting book about relationships is *Love . . . What's Personality Got to Do with It?: Working at Love to Make Love Work*, by Carol Ritberger, Ph.D. (Hay House). Carol uses colors to reflect different personality types: Red is the "get it done" personality (that's me). Orange is the friendly, caring type (that's Gary). Yellow is the creative thinker (which is the color Gary uses to come up with unique ways to help people), and Green is the imaginative, intuitive person who's full of ideas (that's the color I use when doing my medical-intuitive work).

Carol uses various fascinating psychological models, such as the Myers-Briggs formula, to help us understand the role that personality plays in finding, creating, and sustaining loving relationships. (Please visit: **www. ritberger.com**.)

Living from Your Heart

If you've decided to get to the summit of your mountain and not just hang around base camp, then know that ascending to the highest level of living is going to involve your heart. Take a second to check how it's doing right now: Put your hand on your heart and ask, "Is my 'love tap' flowing inside of me?"

You see, we all have a small but powerful golden tap inside of us—while it might be covered over and obscured by leaves and twigs, it's still there. Get to know it, and check in with it on a daily (even hourly) basis. Is your tap turned on enough so that the love from your heart is flowing out to everyone you meet?

I'd like you to read a wonderful little story called *Sara, Book 1: The Foreverness of Friends of a Feather,* by Esther and Jerry Hicks (Hay House). You know Esther—she's the special and pure communicator of the Abraham material, and she and Jerry wrote *Ask and It Is Given: Learning to Manifest Your Desires* (Hay House), a fantastic introduction to the Law of Attraction. The Sara book is a heartwarming tale about a little girl who discovers the secret of creating a happy life; that is, keeping that love spout turned on. Just like Sara, it's time for you to imagine a new way to think and feel that's deep within you and centered from the heart.

The heart is wise, as it knows and feels, and it can't be fooled. Even though you may be taxed and burdened by a life that can be fraught with many disappointments, you can still love. Every night before you go to bed, it helps to examine the day and review your thoughts and actions to find how they could be more loving. Ultimately, when you leave this plane of existence, that's what's going to count.

In order to reach the summit of your own personal mountain, your mandate must be to love, inspire, and serve others in whatever you do—not in some lofty purpose "over there," but in your daily life, right where you are right now.

Three Loving Techniques

Julie Anderson's book, *The Heart: The Final Destination* (I CAN Publishing), seeks to provide insights, inspiration, and guidance about loving more. (Please visit: **www.destinationheart.com**.) With Julie's permission, here are three techniques (in italics) to help open your heart center:

1. Welcome everyone with love. With everyone, including animals, I meet, I automatically say to them mentally, "I welcome you into my life with love." This technique has diffused so many situations I have been confronted with over the years. It puts out an energy and feeling of peace and understanding, whether the other individual knows it or not. When we come from this space of welcoming with love, we are accepting of everyone, no matter who they are or what space they are in. It is the language of the heart.

Like Julie, whenever I meet someone, I always know that he or she is bringing me the next step. I stay aware, listen, and offer a greeting, knowing that out of his or her mouth will come the next piece of information that I need to know. Everything is connected—for many years, I've known that this is how life works. I bring something into the life of each person I meet, and vice versa. This is a loving, positive exchange.

2. Listen to others. Truly listen with your undivided attention when someone is trying to convey something to you. Then repeat back what you think was said. These two techniques not only clarify the information you are receiving but allow you to truly understand where an individual is coming from. So much of our communication between individuals is misunderstood. Listen with the heart into what someone is actually saying, as it may not at all be what you thought you heard. When you are a good listener, others will gravitate to you because they know you love and value them. Sometimes all we need is someone to really hear us and understand us.

Julie gives us great wisdom here. I remember many years ago when one of my daughter's school friends was killed in a car accident. Even though my daughter was a young woman at the time, this dramatic accident affected her deeply—she realized that life is precious and that any one of us could be taken at any time. A few days after the funeral, which was attended by hundreds of young people and their families, my daughter ran into an old employer of hers. Although their working relationship had been less than harmonious, this was an important time for my daughter to appreciate this woman, to focus on and listen to her, and to make this encounter special. Who knew when they might meet again? It's at moments like this that we must be cognizant of the fragility of life.

3. Breathe in love and breathe out blessings. Make this a continual mantra throughout your day. This is a technique I start my day with and continually repeat. It reminds me to think well of others. Remember there is no time or space, and every time you say this you are actually emanating blessings and love to everyone and everything around you.

This actually creates an energy field emanating from your heart like a beacon. Every second of every day, you always have a choice of how to be and how to react to any situation. Pick your choices well and bring harmony to all.

When it comes to breathing, I've personally enjoyed the work of the Vietnamese Zen master Thich Nhat Hanh. His books are filled with the central themes of peace, love, and compassion; and he teaches the art of mindful living and embracing our own reality, which can be tough to do when we're dealing with the effects of this world.

Thich Nhat Hanh has several beautiful meditation CDs, and I love the sound of his peaceful, healing voice. In one of them, he says that we should breathe in the flower, and breathe out freshness. I try to think of that when my mind is in a whirl and I'm trying to do too many things at once. (Please visit: **www.plumvillage. org.**)

My Inspiration for You

For those of us mature folks, staying centered, living from the heart, and breathing in peace and harmony bring us a level of awareness that few youths possess. I believe that diseases begin when we disregard the messages of the heart and deny what gives us happiness— good things will come if we live in joy, harmony, and gratitude.

Regardless of the higher aspects that we strive for, I'm dismayed to see countless people who still completely disregard the physical body. They have terrible diets, rarely exercise, entertain negative thoughts, and hang on to old emotional baggage. I hope that this won't be your path, but that you'll instead do the following:

- Remember the four secrets of vibrant aging—stop the body breakdown, regenerate and repair the body, balance hormones, and ignite your passion.

- Review the layers of physical health—your appearance, your structure, your supply lines, your circulation, your waste systems, and your energy.

- Call in the four alignments of Moses, Buddha, Christ, and Mary to help you to realign with your health and life-purpose goals.

- Finally, use the four powers of creativity—power, vastness, creativity, and deep peace—to aid you in bringing forth your unique gifts before it's too late.

Through any personal health challenge, the miracle of the body still prevails. With a little help, it knows what to do and can repair at any age—I've seen it happen countless times. When the body repairs, the energy returns, the lights go on, the vitality pours back in, and everything lines up! Then emotions take on a rational perspective and spirituality is aligned; thus, we witness the true miracle of the connection between the body, mind, and spirit.

I believe that we can slow down the aging process at this particular point in our history, and that there are tools available for us to do so. Because we're living longer, it behooves us to find these tools and use them. But our highest level of mastery is going to be our personal spiritual evolution—the perfection of our soul.

This brings us to the art of surrender, or the top of the mountain—that is, when you can accept, allow, and enjoy the mystery of life as it unfolds and then ends. My husband, Gary, says that it's a privilege to be with people as they die. He considers it his purpose as a nurse to use his love, energy, and compassion to help his patients transition from one level of existence into the next. He feels that this progression is a beautiful and courageous act, not something to be feared. When the candle of life goes out, we'll merely return to the source to be reborn again.

It has been my greatest pleasure to write this book and give you the information that can help you feel happy, healthy, and fulfilled as you age vibrantly. I hope that you can look back on the piece of patchwork that you've left on the planet with a sense of pride and accomplishment. And, as you review the life that you've passionately lived, may you be able to say, in the words of the famous French chanteuse Edith Piaf: "Non, je ne regrette rien"—"No, I do not regret anything."

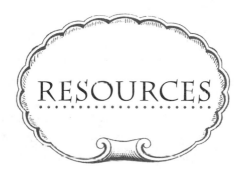

RESOURCES

RECIPES

Fatima's Mint Tea

- Place one large sprig of fresh mint in a clear glass mug.

- Add boiling water and ¼ tsp honey.

- Let steep for a few minutes, and then enjoy the beautiful and vibrant green color, along with the taste. (**Note:** Mint is very useful for the digestion.)

Caroline's Famous Turkey Soup

After Thanksgiving and other holidays, my children always asked me for turkey soup. But you don't need a holiday to make this soup—do so at any time! (**Note:** In place of barley, you may use rice; and in place of turkey, feel free to use chicken.)

- Remove meat from a turkey carcass and set aside. Choose organic where possible. Cover the carcass with water and boil for 2 hours. Remove and discard the carcass; reserve the liquid and meat pieces.

- In a very large pot, sauté 2 large leeks in 3 Tbsp turkey fat or olive oil. Add 4 chopped celery stalks and 2 chopped carrots.

- Add turkey stock, 2 vegetable-bouillon cubes or pan drippings from roasted turkey (remove fat first), and additional water if needed. Add ½ cup barley.

- Simmer until vegetables are tender and barley is soft—about 1 hour. Add reserved turkey meat, a dash of lemon juice, salt and pepper, and serve.

Beef Broth

This recipe has been especially useful for many of my clients:

- Purchase a large bag of organic and hormone-free beef bones, choosing those with some meat left on them. Beef ribs or rib bones work nicely.

- Put the bones on a baking sheet or in a shallow roasting pan, and bake at 325 degrees for about 2 hours.

- Remove the bones from the oven, place in a large pot, cover with water and boil on a *low simmer* for another 2 hours. Strain and drink the broth.

- The purpose of first baking the bones is to remove fat and enhance the flavor of the broth. But for added taste, add a quartered onion or a carrot to the roasting bones. These can be boiled in the pot later with the bones. Salt may be added, too, if so desired.

Drink as much of the broth as you like. When people are weak or very ill, I recommend approximately four to six cups per day. The broth may also be consumed as a beverage, along with regular meals.

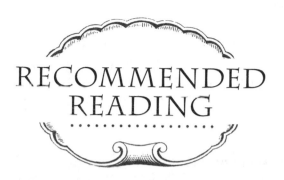

RECOMMENDED READING

Hormone Balancing

Ageless, by Suzanne Somers

Dr. Susan Lark's Hormone Revolution, by Susan Lark, M.D.

HRT—the Answers, by Pamela Wartian Smith, M.D.

Natural Hormone Balance for Women, by Uzzi Reiss, M.D., with Martin Zucker

Safe Estrogen, by Dr. Edward Conley

The Testosterone Syndrome, by Eugene Shippen, M.D., and William Fryer

What Your Doctor May Not Tell You about Menopause, by John R. Lee, M.D., with Virginia Hopkins

You've Hit Menopause, Now What? by George Gillson, M.D., Ph.D., and Tracy Marsden, BScPharm

Vibrant Aging

Chasing Life, by Sanjay Gupta, M.D.

Healthy Aging, by Andrew Weil, M.D.

Younger You, by Eric R. Braverman, M.D.

Health

Healing 101, by Theresa Ramsey, N.M.D.

Protein Power, by Michael R. Eades, M.D., and Mary Dan Eades, M.D.

The Rosedale Diet, by Ron Rosedale, M.D.
Stupid Reasons People Die, by John Corso, M.D.
The 24-Hour Pharmacist, by Suzy Cohen, R.Ph.
The Yeast Connection Handbook, by William G. Crook, M.D.

Personal Empowerment

Finding Your Own North Star, by Martha Beck
From Onions to Pearls, by Satyam Nadeen
Inspiration, by Dr. Wayne W. Dyer
Instant Happiness with the Energy Exchange, by Eve Brinton
Life after Death, by Deepak Chopra, M.D.
Loving What Is, by Byron Katie, with Stephen Mitchell
The Power of Now, by Eckhart Tolle
The Tibetan Book of Living and Dying, by Sogyal Rinpoche
You Can Heal Your Life, by Louise L. Hay
Your Destiny Switch, by Peggy McColl

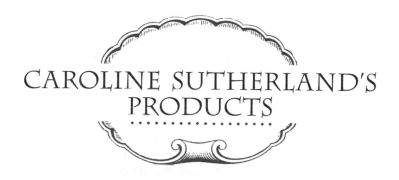

CAROLINE SUTHERLAND'S PRODUCTS

Books

The Body "Knows": How to Tune In to Your Body and Improve Your Health
A primer for understanding health and developing intuition.
$14.95

The Body "Knows" Diet: Cracking the Weight-Loss Code
(Book and CD set)
Identifies the five components of successful weight loss. $16.95

The Body "Knows" Cookbook
Allergy-free cooking. Delicious meals for the whole family.
$13.95

Mommy, I Hurt . . . Mommy, I Love You
A self-help guide for parents and children. This little book inspires parents to help their children over the "rough spots" in a unique, reassuring way, using the principles of relaxation therapy and creative visualization. $10.00

DVDs

The Body "Knows"
Excerpts from Caroline's speeches and classes. $19.95

The Heart of the Family
This parent-education DVD covers a variety of topics

showing unique ways to strengthen communication
between parent and child and blended family members.
(2 hours) $22.00

CDs

The Body "Knows" about Hormones, 4-CD Set
Four hours of interviews with Caroline and Larry Frieders,
R.Ph., regarding the latest information about bioidentical
hormone balancing. $39.95

Tibetan Power Meditation
This deep, powerful meditation CD aligns you to the awesome majesty of Mount Everest, the vast Tibetan skies,
and the sacred peace of Emerald Lake. Adults (60 minutes)
$19.95

Letting Go of the Past & Moving Forward
Have you ever felt unable to let go of the past? Release old
resentments and grievances with soothing reassurance repeated
nightly. Caroline's restful, encouraging voice gives you the confidence to move forward and the willingness to let go. Soothing
wave background. Adults (60 minutes) $19.95

Fountain of Youth—for Women
Deep relaxation and positive programming for women in all
phases of menopause. This CD really helps with personal motivation, anxiety, and sleeplessness. Soothing wave background.
Adults (60 minutes) $19.95

Fountain of Youth—for Men
Deep relaxation and positive programming for the vibrantly
aging male. This CD helps with motivation, inner strength, and
personal empowerment while promoting deep sleep. Soothing
wave background. Adults (60 minutes) $19.95

Couples—Serenity & Tranquility

This CD works to remove blocks to a loving, healthy relationship. In a few short weeks, experience a deeper level of joy and bonding with your loved one and with yourself. Soothing wave background. Adults (60 minutes) $19.95

Body Alive—Deep Relaxation & Sleep

You're guided through a series of phrases about health, immunity, weight control, and abundant energy, as well as improving sleep—great for insomniacs. Soothing, positive wave sounds. Adults (60 minutes) $19.95

Overcoming Jet Lag, Travel Fatigue, or Fear of Flying

A very effective CD, recommended by travelers, flight attendants, pilots, and businesspeople for jet lag and fear of flying. Soothing wave background. Adults (60 minutes) $19.95

Meditation & Music

A relaxing guided-meditation CD designed to center you, focus the breath, work with your own affirmations, and help access that deep state of peace within you. This CD is set to beautiful music, created by award-winning musician Paul Armitage. Adults (60 minutes) $19.95

Motivation & Confidence for Teenagers & Young People

Parents say this CD can put the *terrific* back into your teenager. In three to four weeks of nightly listening, teenagers can expect to feel an increase in self-esteem, motivation, and positive choices. Soothing wave background. Adolescents ages 12 and over (60 minutes) $19.95

Ace Those Exams!

Decreases the fear and anxiety of exams, while increasing memory and mental ability. Really works for teens *and* adults! Soothing wave background. Adults and adolescents, ages 12 and over (60 minutes) $19.95

Children's Products

My Little Angel Gift Sets

Welcome to the world of Angels 4 Kids®—angels, CDs, and story-books that reassure and encourage children. All sets include a soft, cuddly angel, which is handmade and machine washable in soft cotton velour, and a positive, uplifting 60-minute story/music CD. Angels come with white or ethnic (brown) faces and are suitable for both boys and girls, ages toddler to teenager.

— *My Little Angel Tells Me I'm Special®.* This story helps children fall asleep and build self-esteem. A general CD that's useful for all children—babies to 10 years (adults and teens love them, too). Cost per angel set: $24.95

— *My Little Angel Helps Me and My Family®.* This story supports and comforts children who are adjusting to a family breakup, separation, or divorce. Cost per angel set: $24.95

— *My Little Angel Helps Me in the Hospital®.* This story calms, comforts, and reassures children who require hospitalization for major or minor surgery, serious illness, cancer treatment, burns, or any surgical procedure. Cost per angel set: $24.95

— *My Little Angel Loves Me®.* This story reassures, comforts, and supports children (and adults) who have been abused, traumatized, or mistreated. Cost per angel set: $24.95

Body Alive (Children)—Confidence & Self-Esteem CD

Helps your child understand body processes, as well as developing a healthy attitude about food choices, physical activity, confidence, and positive values. Set to beautiful music. Ages 3–10 (60 minutes) $19.95

School Work & Making Friends CD

Helps develop love and excitement about school and learning, as well as helping the child overcome blocks and barriers to playing and sharing with others. Set to enchanting music. Ages 3–10 (60 minutes) $19.95

The Changing Family—Feeling Safe and Secure CD
Helps reassure and comfort children in a changing family situation such as a divorce or separation. Ages 3–10 (60 minutes) $19.95

For a complete listing of all of Caroline Sutherland's
products and seminars, visit:
www.carolinesutherland.com or
www.angels4kids.com

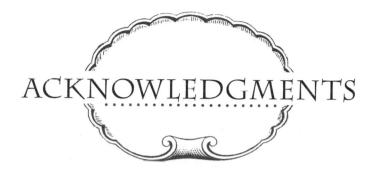

ACKNOWLEDGMENTS

This book would not have been possible without the support and encouragement of my mentor and publisher, Louise Hay, and the entire Hay House team. It has been my pleasure to be a Hay House author since 1999—as a writer, this opportunity has given me the platform to spread the message that the body knows what to do at any age, and that vibrant health is not a mystery.

I'm grateful to my husband, Gary; my daughters, Jennifer and Erica; and my wonderful family and many friends, whose constant faith and interest propel me forward to fulfill my destiny as a health educator and medical intuitive.

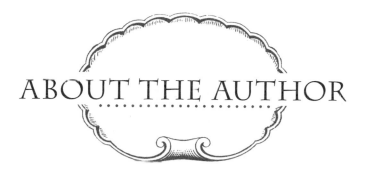

ABOUT THE AUTHOR

Caroline Sutherland has a vast clinical background as an allergy-testing technician in environmental medicine, where her intuitive gift developed. She was raised in a medical family in which both her father and grandfather were medical doctors. As a child, the "blueprint" of her family lineage created important seeds for her future career as a medical intuitive. For more than 25 years, she has lectured internationally on the subject, and her intuitive impressions have positively impacted the lives of more than 100,000 people.

Caroline is the author of numerous books and audio programs on health, personal development, and self-esteem; as well as the founder of Sutherland Communications, which offers medical-intuitive training, weight-loss programs, and consultation services for adults and children. She is a popular guest on radio and television.

Website: **www.carolinesutherland.com**

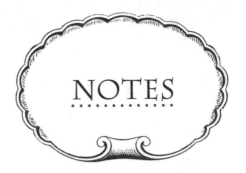

NOTES

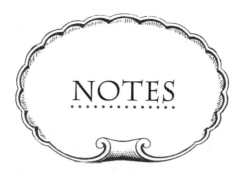

NOTES

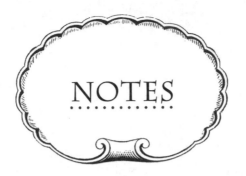

NOTES

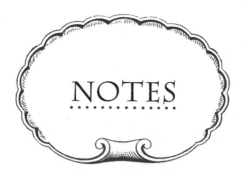

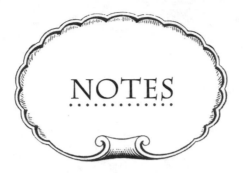

NOTES

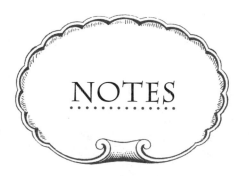

NOTES

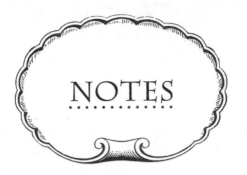

NOTES

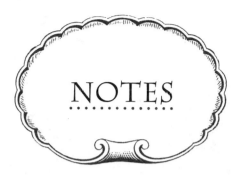

NOTES

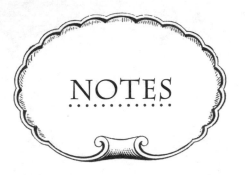

NOTES

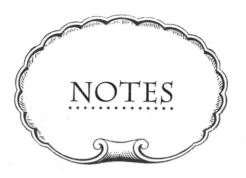

NOTES

We hope you enjoyed this Hay House book. If you'd like to receive a free catalog featuring additional Hay House books and products, or if you'd like information about the Hay Foundation, please contact:

Hay House, Inc.
P.O. Box 5100
Carlsbad, CA 92018-5100

(760) 431-7695 or **(800) 654-5126**
(760) 431-6948 (fax) or **(800) 650-5115 (fax)**
www.hayhouse.com® • **www.hayfoundation.org**

Published and distributed in Australia by: Hay House Australia Pty. Ltd., 18/36 Ralph St., Alexandria NSW 2015 • *Phone:* 612-9669-4299 *Fax:* 612 9669-4144 • www.hayhouse.com.au

Published and distributed in the United Kingdom by: Hay House UK, Ltd., 292B Kensal Rd., London W10 5BE • *Phone:* 44-20-8962-1230 • *Fax:* 44-20-8962-1239 • www.hayhouse.co.uk

Published and distributed in the Republic of South Africa by: Hay House SA (Pty), Ltd., P.O. Box 990, Witkoppen 2068 • *Phone/Fax:* 27-11-467-8904 • orders@psdprom.co.za • www.hayhouse.co.za

Published in India by: Hay House Publishers India, Muskaan Complex, Plot No. 3, B-2, Vasant Kunj, New Delhi 110 070 • *Phone:* 91-11-4176-1620 • *Fax:* 91-11-4176-1630 • www.hayhouse.co.in

Distributed in Canada by: Raincoast, 9050 Shaughnessy St., Vancouver, B.C. V6P 6E5 • *Phone:* (604) 323-7100 *Fax:* (604) 323-2600 • www.raincoast.com

Tune in to **HayHouseRadio.com®** for the best in inspirational talk radio featuring top Hay House authors! And, sign up via the Hay House USA Website to receive the Hay House online newsletter and stay informed about what's going on with your favorite authors. You'll receive bimonthly announcements about Discounts and Offers, Special Events, Product Highlights, Free Excerpts, Giveaways, and more! **www.hayhouse.com®**